Clinical Handbook of Neuromuscular Medicine

T0171953

David Walk

Editor

Clinical Handbook
of Neuromuscular Medicine

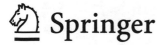 Springer

Editor
David Walk
Department of Neurology
University of Minnesota
Minneapolis, MN, USA

ISBN 978-3-030-09791-2   ISBN 978-3-319-67116-1   (eBook)
https://doi.org/10.1007/978-3-319-67116-1

Printed on acid-free paper

This Springer imprint is published by the registered company Springer International Publishing AG
part of Springer Nature
The registered company address is: Gewerbestrasse 11, 6330 Cham, Switzerland

Foreword

The neuromuscular specialists at the University of Minnesota Medical Center have made a significant contribution to the literature on diseases of the nerve and muscle. Students of neuromuscular disorders will appreciate this concise and targeted approach to the basic information needed to deal with such a patient. Each chapter begins with key points that are emphasized in the short chapters to follow. Early exposure to some of these pearls of neuromuscular knowledge is essential to the learning process. For example, in the chapter on diseases of muscle, one of the key points is "not every high CK is due to myopathy." How true! Another chapter on disorders of neuromuscular transmission emphatically states: "Prednisone remains the cornerstone of MG immunotherapy"—again, a critical teaching point that many physicians have trouble accepting, so very much a key point worth emphasizing. The concise chapters after the key point introductions are again to the point and without speculation, theory, or basic science details. The chapters are ultimately *practical* and *useful* sources of reconstruction for the practicing clinician. Tables are easy to read. References are left to a minimum and just enough to be useful. Therefore, despite the concise brevity of this book, it is loaded with information that if actually learned will allow a physician to be able to provide expert care for a patient with a neuromuscular disorder. Indeed, Dr. Walk in his preface boldly says the goal of his group was to provide a book that could be read in a weekend. They have effectively done this. Dr. Walk also says that while the volume is probably most appropriate for neuromuscular fellows, perhaps a non-neurologist forced to care for a neuromuscular patient may find some approaches that can be taken until the patient can get in to see a neuromuscular specialist. I enjoy David's candid and honest statements like these because they again are shockingly true.

I believe neuromuscular fellows and other health-care providers needing to care for a patient with a neuromuscular disorder will benefit greatly from this brief handbook.

Richard J. Barohn, MD
Gertrude and Dewey Professor of Neurology
University Distinguished Professor
President Research Institute
Vice Chancellor for Research
University of Kansas Medical Center
Kansas City, Kansas

Preface

I've often said that among all nonsurgical specialties, primary care providers are least comfortable managing neurological problems and that among all neurological subspecialties, neurologists are least comfortable managing neuromuscular problems. To the extent that this may be true, it may reflect deficiencies in medical education. In the United States, where I have trained and worked until now, clinical neurology is sometimes optional, and rarely emphasized, in undergraduate medical education. Because neurology is not considered a subspecialty of internal medicine, specialists in internal medicine have less direct exposure to neurologists than to colleagues specializing in diseases of other organ systems. The problem may be confounded by the amusing but insidious lay perception that understanding the organ responsible for intelligence must, *a priori*, require superior intelligence compared to, say, understanding the organs responsible for excretion.

As for neurologists' perception of neuromuscular medicine, this problem too may be a consequence of deficiencies in medical education. Postgraduate training in neurology in the United States currently involves an inordinate amount of time spent in hospitals, while neurologic *practice* does not. As a result trainees in neurology quickly become competent at managing acute stroke, encephalopathy, and status epilepticus but are often baffled by the most common neuropathies. This front-loading of training in acute neurological problems also biases trainees' choice of mentors and fellowships and as noted prepares them poorly for careers in general neurology.

This book is designed to address these problems. Our target audience is postgraduate trainees in neurology, principally neurology residents or those starting a fellowship in neuromuscular medicine, but to borrow a phrase from houses of worship, all are welcome. Perhaps an orthopedic surgeon interested in a better understanding of causes of leg weakness will seek guidance here, or a rural practitioner who, realizing that the nearest neurologist is far away and has no openings for months, would like to learn more to help their patients with nerve and muscle disease.

As for our tactical approach, it is as follows: *we believe the best way to achieve our objective is to deliver all the essential information in neuromuscular medicine in a book that can be read in a weekend.* If you read this whole book and are reasonably attentive while doing so, you will have a framework for the approach to neuromuscular diagnosis and management and will have read, at least once, everything you need to know if you are in our target audience.

At least, that's our goal. We hope we succeed. Thanks for choosing to learn about this extraordinary subspecialty.

I would like to acknowledge and thank Ben Bornzstein, Ph.D., for his help and encouragement, my co-authors, for their patience and commitment, and my wife, Missy Walk, for her guidance and wisdom.

Minneapolis, MN, USA   David Walk, MD

Contents

Contributors

Jeffrey A. Allen, MD University of Minnesota, Department of Neurology, Minneapolis, MN, USA

Matthew Bower, MS University of Minnesota Health, Department of Genetic Counseling, Minneapolis, MN, USA

Deanna Diebold, MD University of Minnesota, Pulmonary, Critical Care, and Sleep Medicine, Minneapolis, MN, USA

Peter I. Karachunski, MD University of Minnesota, Department of Neurology, Minneapolis, MN, USA

Georgios Manousakis, MD University of Minnesota, Department of Neurology, Minneapolis, MN, USA

Robin Samuel, OTR/L University of Minnesota Health, Fairview Rehabilitation Services, Minneapolis, MN, USA

David Walk, MD University of Minnesota, Department of Neurology, Minneapolis, MN, USA

Chapter 1
Introduction

David Walk

Neuromuscular disease is a term applied to conditions of nerve roots, axons, the neuromuscular junction, and muscle. Disorders of motor neurons, dorsal root ganglia, cranial nerve nuclei, and autonomic ganglia and axons are generally considered in this category as well. Hence, neuromuscular diseases typically present *with* at least one of the following:

- Weakness
- Loss of sensation
- Abnormal sensation

and *without* any of the following:

- Cognitive or higher cortical dysfunction
- Abnormal involuntary movements
- Bradykinesia or rigidity
- Pathologic reflexes or spasticity
- A sensory level

Of course, this concept is tidy but inaccurate. The obvious exception is the presence of spastic dysarthria, hyperreflexia, and spasticity in primary lateral sclerosis and amyotrophic lateral sclerosis (ALS), conditions typically managed in neuromuscular medicine clinics; however, advances in our understanding of neuromuscular diseases have also identified other examples of central nervous system pathology associated with conditions traditionally categorized as neuromuscular. Examples again include ALS, which is often associated with cognitive impairment, behavioral impairment, or frontotemporal dementia; myotonic dystrophy, a multi-system disorder often associated with cognitive dysfunction and central sleep disorders; and mitochondrial disorders, which can have broad consequences in muscle, central

D. Walk, MD (✉)
University of Minnesota, Department of Neurology, Minneapolis, MN, USA
e-mail: walkx001@umn.edu

© Springer International Publishing AG, part of Springer Nature 2018
D. Walk (ed.), *Clinical Handbook of Neuromuscular Medicine*,
https://doi.org/10.1007/978-3-319-67116-1_1

nervous system, and other organ systems. Furthermore, many chief complaints have a broad differential diagnosis that includes neuromuscular and musculoskeletal disorders. Our rapidly expanding knowledge of neuromuscular genetics has also identified unexpected genotype-phenotype associations. Hence, the neuromuscular diagnostician must be careful to not prejudge the diagnosis before obtaining the rich dataset available in a comprehensive medical history and examination.

Clinical Assessment of Suspected Neuromuscular Disease

Neurologists teach trainees that neurologic diagnosis hinges on three questions:

- *Is this a neurologic disorder?*
- *If it is, what is the anatomic localization?*
- *Based upon the history and anatomic localization, what are the most likely pathologic diagnoses?*

In reality, much of neurologic practice relies heavily on recognizing pathognomonic presentations, such as migraine, essential tremor, or absence seizures. In neuromuscular medicine, however, this structured and logical diagnostic paradigm is still the key to accurate diagnosis. For those who appreciate its unyielding logic and reliance on accurate data collection, this is one of the great appeals of this subspecialty. This introduction focuses on the art of the neuromuscular history and examination.

The Neuromuscular Medical History

Turning a Chief Complaint into a Localization Hypothesis

The objective of neuromuscular history-taking is to turn a chief complaint into a hypothesis regarding localization. The objective of the neurologic examination is to test that hypothesis. In evaluating the chief complaint, it is critical to ask clarifying questions relentlessly until one or more localizations emerge as most likely. Here are some important rules when assessing the chief complaint:

- *If the chief complaint is "weakness," find out what the functional disability is. Ask, "what do you have difficulty doing?"*
- *If the chief complaint is "numbness," find out what in fact is perceived. Is this a spontaneous abnormal sensation, a loss of sensation, or weakness described as numbness?*
- *If the chief complaint is pain, ask about pain descriptors (aching, burning, shooting, etc.), whether it is deep or superficial ("does it feel like it's in the skin, muscle, or bone?") and whether there is associated allodynia or hyperalgesia.*

- *If the chief complaint is pain, find out if it is worst with <u>use of the limb or weight bearing</u>, as is often the case with musculoskeletal conditions, or <u>at rest</u>, which is common with neuropathic pain.*
- *Ask about cranial symptoms in all pure motor syndromes.*
- *Ask about muscle cramps in all pure motor syndromes.*

Other important things to remember in the neuromuscular history include the following:

- *Social history*

  - *Ask about alcohol use, occupational, and recreational exposures so as not to miss a toxic etiology.*
  - *Find out your patient's occupation and family circumstances, as many neuro-muscular disorders disproportionately impact activities of daily living and instrumental activities of daily living and require work accommodations, dis-ability determination, or help with caregiving.*

- *Family history*

  - *Construct a family tree and include parents, children, aunts, uncles, and grandparents. Ask broadly about neurologic and psychiatric disorders and not only the patient's chief complaint, as some pathogenic mutations can present with a wide variety of syndromes. Find out at what age people died. "Family history is negative" is not sufficient.*

- *Review of systems*

  - *Certain chief complaints mandate learning about certain systems.*

    - *Suspected muscular dystrophy: cardiac ROS*
    - *Suspected inflammatory disease: rheumatologic ROS*

The Neuromuscular Examination

The goal of the neurologic examination is to test the localization hypotheses (differential diagnosis) established by the history. Hence the standard neurologic examination represents a framework which is supplemented by aspects that are best positioned to test those hypotheses.

- *Mental status*

  - *The mental status examination is of limited importance when considering many neuromuscular conditions; however some, such as ALS and myotonic dystrophy, can be associated with executive dysfunction.*

- *Cranial nerves*

  - *Ptosis and weakness of extraocular muscles are prevalent in mitochondrial disorders, oculopharyngeal muscular dystrophy, and myasthenia gravis, among other conditions.*
  - *Facial weakness is prevalent in myasthenia gravis, spinobulbar muscular atrophy, and ALS, among other conditions. Orbicularis oculi strength can be tested with manual muscle testing, using the examiner's fingers to overcome forceful eye closure. Orbicularis oris strength can be tested by asking the patient to puff out their cheeks fully.*
  - *Bulbar examination is critical when evaluating for oculopharyngeal muscular dystrophy, myasthenia gravis, and motor neuron disorders.*

    - Bulbar upper motor neuron signs *include a strained, strangled speech quality; slow repetitive articulation of labial ("pa"), lingual ("ta"), and guttural ("ka") sounds; and slow side-to-side tongue movements. An exaggerated gag reflex, brisk masseter reflex, and pseudobulbar affect are commonly present with these.*
    - Bulbar lower motor neuron signs *include weakness of facial muscles, breathy speech quality, tongue atrophy, tongue fasciculations, and tongue weakness, tested by asking the patient to press the tongue against the inside of the cheek and attempting to overcome this with the examiner's finger placed outside the cheek. A weak tongue will not elevate the cheek and will often protrude anteriorly when this is attempted.*

  - Neck weakness *is prevalent in numerous neuromuscular conditions.*

    - Neck extension *relies principally on cervical paraspinal muscles and can be weak in a wide range of neuromuscular conditions including high cervical radiculopathy, inflammatory myopathy, axial myopathy, and ALS.*
    - Neck flexion *relies heavily on the sternocleidomastoid muscles and is often weak in ALS. The sternocleidomastoid muscles can also be tested individually.*

- *Sensory examination*

  - *Screening: if a pure motor condition is suspected, screening for sensory involvement can be limited to testing distal extremities for touch, pin, and vibratory sensation.*
  - *Sensory or sensorimotor conditions*

    - Tactile perception *can be tested objectively by touching gently with cotton and asking the patient to identify the area touched with eyes closed.*
    - Small-fiber modalities*: Perception of sharpness is usually easier to test and more reliable than temperature; temperature can be used as an adjunct if pin testing provides surprising results.*

      - *First, test an area likely to be normal, based upon the history. If possible, establish that as normal sharpness, and then test the symptomatic area. If perception of sharpness is reduced in the symptomatic area, identify the margins of the affected area by testing radially or proximally in the case of a length-dependent presentation, until sharp sensation is normal or nearly normal.*

- *Note abnormal sensory phenomena, such as a delay in the perception of sharpness or hyperalgesia.*

- Large-fiber modalities: *Vibratory sense perception is a more sensitive indicator than position sense.*

  - *Quantify vibratory sense deficits using timed vibration with a standard 128 Hz tuning fork or vibration scores using a Rydell-Seiffer tuning fork [1]. In a length-dependent process, begin with distal-most sites and move proximally until vibration is perceived or is normal. Test each site 2–3 times to establish consistent scores.*
  - *Some people with profound sensory loss or positive sensory symptoms will report vibration when none is present (positive responses to null stimuli). Always test with null stimuli at least once (apply a tuning fork that is not vibrating with patient's eyes closed). If positive responses to null stimuli are reported, train the patient to recognize the difference in a sensate region. If they still have difficulty, use a forced-choice algorithm, in which two stimuli are applied, one vibrating and one not, to determine whether the patient can correctly and reproducibly distinguish vibration from pressure.*
  - *A forced-choice algorithm can also be helpful when examining people with slow reaction times, as the standard method of limits testing is reaction time-dependent.*
  - *Testing of position sense is usually not necessary unless a profound loss of vibratory sense is noted.*

- *Motor examination consists of testing tone, bulk, and strength. Testing all three is critical in neuromuscular disease. Exposing the limbs is necessary to evaluate bulk.*

  - Tone: *Passive stretch can identify reduced tone, spasticity, rigidity, or paratonia. All are localizing: reduced tone indicates nerve or muscle disease, spasticity indicates disease of motor neurons or their axons (corticospinal tract), rigidity indicates extrapyramidal disease, and paratonia indicates premotor frontal lobe disease. While testing tone, inspect the limb for atrophy, fasciculations, and signs of musculoskeletal or vascular conditions.*
  - Bulk: *Neurogenic atrophy is easy to identify and is a critically valuable objective sign.*
  - Strength

    - *Be sure to use the Medical Research Council (MRC) scale [2] correctly. Normal strength for a patient's habitus and medical condition should be scored 5, even if they are relatively weak compared to larger or healthier patients. Use 4+, 4, and 4- to indicate force generation against strong, moderate, or minimal resistance but avoid further gradations as they are poorly reproducible. Position the limb appropriately with respect to gravity to test scores of 3 or 2, and assign those scores only if the patient can move the limb throughout its range of motion.*

- *Identify a set of muscle groups that you examine routinely, and deviate from that routine only when relevant to the localization hypothesis. For example, testing strength of finger flexors is not useful in most circumstances but is critical when considering inclusion body myositis.*
- *Test each muscle group without preconceptions. A common mistake made by inexperienced examiners is to erroneously score all muscle groups at 4 when they anticipate weakness based upon the history. If you score each muscle group accurately, you will identify common patterns that establish the localization. A score of 4 in all muscle groups never occurs because pathology follows characteristic patterns of weakness.*
- *Score impersistent resistance, or "giveaway," based upon the force initially generated, no matter how briefly. Giveaway usually reflects severe sensory loss or inadequate effort rather than pathology of motor neuron, neuromuscular junction, or muscle, and downgrading the MRC score due to giveaway will lead to an erroneous diagnosis.*

- *Reflexes: The normal range is broad, from trace to 3+ with spread. Consider the following pearls:*

  - *Check the masseter reflex ("jaw jerk"). A brisk jaw jerk indicates that limb hyperreflexia is due to cranial, rather than cervical, disease and can also be an upper motor neuron sign in ALS.*
  - *Record reflex spread. While this can be normal, it is an indicator of relative hyperreflexia and should increase one's suspicion for the presence of corticospinal tract disease.*
  - *Take note of findings that are in the normal range but discount the localization hypothesis, such as brisk Achilles reflexes in a person with suspected polyneuropathy.*
  - *An absent reflex in a non-paralyzed muscle usually indicates dysfunction of the afferent, rather than the efferent, limb of the reflex arc.*

- *Coordination: Note the nature of abnormalities when present (e.g., action tremor or dysmetria). Remember that slowing of rapid repetitive or rapid alternating movements is a sensitive sign of corticospinal tract dysfunction.*
- *Gait and station: Evaluation of gait and station is critical in neuromuscular disease, both as a diagnostic tool and an indicator of functional status and safety in independent living. The following are some highly localizing findings in this part of the examination:*

  - *Axial weakness*

    - *Camptocormia*
    - *"Dropped head syndrome"*

- *Proximal weakness*

  - *Difficulty standing from a kneeling, crouching, or seating position*
  - *Exaggerated lumbar lordosis while walking*
  - *Exaggerated truncal sway while walking*
  - *Trendelenburg gait*

- *Knee extension weakness*

  - *"Locking" knees into hyperextension while walking*

- *Length-dependent polyneuropathy*

  - *Steppage gait*
  - *Inability to stand or walk on heels*

- *Miyoshi myopathy*

  - *Inability to stand or walk on toes*

- *Severe large fiber sensory neuropathy*

  - *Inability to maintain stance, even with eyes open*

    - *Easier while walking*
    - *Much easier when gently touching wall or furniture*

  - *Inability to maintain stance with eyes closed*

As you perform the history and examination, keep the following question in mind: *are the findings concordant*? While performing a history and physical examination, a novice examiner commonly gathers a list of facts that, upon reflection, point in disparate directions. As you gain skill in this field, you will find yourself honing a differential diagnosis as you go, revisiting statements or findings that are not concordant with others and finishing with a moderate or high level of confidence regarding the presence or absence of neurologic disease and, if present, the likely anatomic localization.

Confirmation of the anatomic localization can often be obtained with electrodiagnostic testing. Muscle biopsy, genetic testing, and other laboratory studies are generally most helpful in confirming the pathologic process. Experience indicates that the utility of these confirmatory studies correlates closely with the accuracy and specificity of the conclusions reached from the structured neuromuscular history and examination.

References

1. Alanazy MH, Alfurayh NA, Almweisheer SN, Aljafen BN, Muayqil T. The conventional tuning fork as a quantitative tool for vibration threshold. Muscle Nerve 2018;57:49–53.
2. O'Brien, M. *Aids to the Examination of the Peripheral Nervous System*, 5th ed. Edinburgh, 2010.

Chapter 2
Diseases of Muscle

Georgios Manousakis

Abbreviations

AQM	Acute quadriplegic myopathy
CK	Creatine kinase
DM	Dermatomyositis
DM1	Myotonic dystrophy type 1
DM2	Myotonic dystrophy type 2
FSHD	Facioscapularhumeral dystrophy
IBM	Inclusion body myositis
LGMD	Limb girdle muscular dystrophy
MELAS	Mitochondrial myopathy, lactic acidosis, and stroke-like episodes
MERRF	Myoclonic epilepsy and ragged red fibers
MNGIE	Mitochondrial neurogastro-intestinal encephalomyopathy
OPMD	Oculopharyngeal muscular dystrophy
PM	Polymyositis

Key Points
- The most common pattern of weakness in myopathy is proximal, limb-girdle, and symmetric. Other less common patterns are important to recognize, due to their much more restricted differential diagnosis (Table 2.1).
- Timing of development of muscle weakness (acute, subacute versus chronic) can assist in differential diagnosis.
- Myalgia that is not exercise-induced, and not associated with elevated creatine kinase (CK), myopathic EMG, or abnormal clinical muscle examination, is unlikely to be of neuromuscular etiology.
- Not every high CK is due to myopathy.
- Myopathic features on EMG include abnormal spontaneous activity, such as fibrillations or myotonia, and early recruitment of small, short-duration, polyphasic motor unit potentials.

G. Manousakis, MD (✉)
University of Minnesota, Department of Neurology, Minneapolis, MN, USA
e-mail: gmanousa@umn.edu

© Springer International Publishing AG, part of Springer Nature 2018
D. Walk (ed.), *Clinical Handbook of Neuromuscular Medicine*,
https://doi.org/10.1007/978-3-319-67116-1_2

- Open or needle muscle biopsy allows morphometric, histochemical, biochemical, genetic, and electron microscopic analysis of muscle and remains one of the most valuable tools in the diagnosis of myopathy.
- Muscle imaging with ultrasound and/or MRI allows noninvasive assessment of general category of muscle pathology, recognition of patterns of muscle involvement with limited differential diagnosis, and assists in guiding choice of muscle for biopsy.
- Forearm exercise test assesses the rise in lactate and ammonia after maximal isometric exercise and is helpful in the diagnosis of dynamic glycogen storage disorders such as McArdle disease and myoadenylate deaminase deficiency.
- Some muscular dystrophies and congenital myopathies, particularly RYR1 mutations, are associated with an increased risk of malignant hyperthermia or rhabdomyolysis after exposure to inhalational anesthetic agents. Patients with this disorder are advised to share this information with their anesthesiologist before undergoing general anesthesia.
- Duchenne muscular dystrophy (DMD) is the most common muscular dystrophy, occurring in 1:3500 male births. It is X-linked and due to dystrophin gene mutations. Loss of ambulation typically occurs between age 12 and 14. Cardiomyopathy and respiratory failure occur almost universally in later stages, necessitating regular surveillance since childhood.
- Medications that can alter the natural history of DMD include oral corticosteroids and eteplirsen, a recently approved exon-skipping antisense oligonucleotide therapy for DMD patients with selected mutations.
- Patients with facioscapulohumeral dystrophy (FSHD) present with characteristic asymmetric weakness of scapular, humeral (biceps and triceps, with notable sparing of deltoid), peroneal, and facial muscles.
- Type 1 myotonic dystrophy is the most common adult onset muscular dystrophy (1:10,000 adults). The pattern of weakness is characteristic with atrophy of temporalis, facial muscles, ptosis, frontal balding, handgrip and foot dorsiflexion weakness with prominent myotonia. It is autosomal dominant, and anticipation, with onset of symptoms earlier in subsequent generations, occurs quite frequently.
- Type 1 myotonic dystrophy is a multisystem disorder causing abnormalities of cardiac conduction; cataracts; excessive daytime sleepiness; gastrointestinal, endocrine, cognitive disorders; and selected neoplasms. Sudden death from cardiac arrhythmia is the leading cause of death, and therefore regular surveillance for the above complications is standard of care.
- Type 2 myotonic dystrophy is harder to recognize than type 1, because the pattern of weakness is proximal, similar to other common myopathies, age of onset is later than type 1, and clinical myotonia is present in <50% of cases.
- Limb-girdle muscular dystrophies are a large and heterogeneous group of dominantly or recessively inherited muscle diseases with variable ages of onset, patterns of muscle weakness, and ethnic group predilection.
- Distal myopathies are a large group of inherited muscle diseases. They are differentiated clinically from a length-dependent neuropathy or motor neuron disease by the relative sparing of intrinsic foot muscles despite atrophy of calf muscles. Selective involvement of anterior versus posterior compartment of the legs can assist in differential diagnosis.

- Oculopharyngeal muscular dystrophy (OPMD) is an adult onset autosomal dominant myopathy that is very prevalent among French Canadians. It manifests with slowly progressive ptosis, ophthalmoparesis, and dysphagia, with onset around age 50.
- The pathognomonic skin rashes of dermatomyositis are the heliotrope sign and the Gottron's papules. Photosensitive skin rash around the neck and nail telangiectasias may also be present.
- Twenty percent or more of dermatomyositis cases occurring over age 40 are paraneoplastic, and an extensive search for underlying malignancy is required in this subset of patients.
- The histologic hallmark findings of dermatomyositis are perifascicular atrophy, vasculopathy, and perivascular or perimysial inflammation.
- Polymyositis (PM) is a rather uncommon disorder, characterized by limb-girdle symmetric muscle weakness, elevated CK, and muscle biopsy showing focal invasion of non-necrotic muscle fibers by lymphocytes. It responds to immunotherapy similar to dermatomyositis.
- Anti-synthetase syndrome is characterized by myositis, interstitial lung disease, nonerosive arthritis, characteristic skin and muscle biopsy changes, and positive anti-synthetase antibodies, with Jo-1 being the most common.
- Selective, asymmetric weakness of long finger flexors and quadriceps is highly characteristic, if not pathognomonic, for inclusion body myositis (IBM). Unlike other inflammatory myopathies, IBM responds poorly to immunotherapy and progresses slowly over years.
- Dysphagia occurs in more than 30% of patients with IBM. Sometimes it may respond to cricopharyngeal myotomy.
- The diagnosis of IBM is confirmed by muscle biopsy. The four cardinal histologic findings are focal invasion of non-necrotic fibers by lymphocytes, rimmed vacuoles, MHC I upregulation, and aggregation of abnormal proteins, including amyloid and p62.
- Serum antibodies against cytosolic nucleotidase 5–1 alpha (NT5C1a IgG) show ~50% sensitivity and 90% specificity for the diagnosis of IBM.
- Immune-mediated necrotizing myopathies produce severe and rapidly progressive limb-girdle weakness with marked CK elevations. They are associated with SRP, HMG-CoA-reductase antibodies, and connective tissue disorders or paraneoplastic syndromes. Aggressive immunotherapy is required.
- Statin-induced myopathy is a heterogeneous term referring to symptoms ranging from myalgias and asymptomatic hyperCKemia, to rhabdomyolysis, and the most severe, and rare, autoimmune necrotizing myopathy with HMG-CoA-reductase antibodies, which requires immunotherapy in addition to statin discontinuation.
- Pompe disease is an autosomal recessive disorder due to deficiency of the acid maltase enzyme. It can present similarly to many childhood or adult onset muscular dystrophies. Early respiratory failure occurring in an ambulatory patient, tongue weakness, and myotonic discharges on EMG are some clues to the diagnosis. The diagnosis is confirmed by measurement of the acid maltase enzyme activity in dried blood spot sample, muscle biopsy, or DNA testing.

- Treatment of Pompe disease includes intravenous recombinant alpha-glucosidase, which can be lifesaving in infants and slows the progression of respiratory failure and weakness in adults.
- McArdle disease is caused by deficiency of muscle phosphorylase. Rhabdomyolysis after short, intense anaerobic exercise and the second wind phenomenon are the distinguishing clinical features.
- Carnitine palmitoyltransferase 2 (CPT2) mutations are the most common metabolic cause of recurrent rhabdomyolysis in adults.
- Myotonia congenita is caused by CLCN1 gene mutations. Muscle stiffness or cramps are the chief complaints. Patients often show prominent muscle hypertrophy, and weakness is minimal to none.
- Paramyotonia congenita and hyperkalemic periodic paralysis are caused by SCN4A gene mutations. The term paramyotonia refers to paradoxical worsening of myotonia following exercise or cold exposure.
- Hypokalemic periodic paralysis is a cause of episodic muscle weakness. High carbohydrate loads and intense exercise are common triggers. Causes include mutations in CACN1A gene, thyrotoxicosis, and secondary causes of hypokalemia.
- Mitochondrial disorders affect multiple organs, including the heart, endocrine glands, retina, muscle, and brain.
- Confirmation of mitochondrial myopathy diagnosis usually requires muscle biopsy, showing ragged red, ragged blue, cytochrome oxidase-negative fibers, or a biochemical defect in complexes I–V or identification of a DNA mutation affecting the mitochondrial machinery, from either muscle tissue or leukocytes.
- Kearns-Sayre syndrome is the triad of progressive external ophthalmoplegia, pigmentary retinopathy, and cardiac conduction defects, with onset typically before age 20.
- MELAS syndrome can present with recurrent stroke in different vascular territories in young individuals. L-arginine treatment can be helpful.
- MERRF is the acronym for myoclonic epilepsy with ragged red fibers. It can mimic juvenile myoclonic epilepsy. Weakness, ataxia, and hearing loss are selected additional features.
- MNGIE syndrome is a mitochondrial disorder characterized by ophthalmoplegia, neuropathy, mimicking CMT or CIDP, leukoencephalopathy, and recurrent intestinal pseudo-obstruction or gastroparesis leading to weight loss and emaciation. Some cases can be treated with bone marrow transplantation.
- Hypothyroidism can cause myalgia, hyperCKemia, proximal weakness, myoedema, and rarely muscle hypertrophy.
- Thyrotoxicosis from Graves' disease causes a restrictive ophthalmoparesis.
- Acute quadriplegic myopathy is the most common neuromuscular cause of weakness and difficulty weaning in intensive care settings. Sepsis and prolonged ICU stay, regardless of corticosteroid exposure, are risk factors. The condition is reversible but recovery occurs very slowly.
- The most common congenital myopathy is central core disease due to autosomal dominant ryanodine receptor-1 (RYR1) mutations. It is associated with high risk of malignant hyperthermia.

General Approach to Myopathies: Symptoms, Clinical Signs, and Diagnostic Evaluation

Myopathies can present with *negative* (weakness, paralysis) or *positive* (myalgia, cramps, myoglobinuria) symptoms. Weakness is the clinical sign of reduced muscle power, measured on the 0–5 Medical Research Council (MRC) scale or, quantitatively, by handheld dynamometry. Report of weakness by the patient without demonstrable reduction of muscle power is often not due to neuromuscular causes.

Myopathic weakness is typically proximal (limb-girdle distribution) and symmetric. This pattern has a vast differential diagnosis, is not specific, and can be also seen in neuromuscular junction disorders such as myasthenia gravis, motor neuron syndromes, or immune-mediated neuropathies.

By contrast, some myopathies have more specific patterns of weakness involving cranial, axial, or distal limb muscles. These are listed in Table 2.1.

Table 2.1 Myopathies presenting with prominent cranial, axial, or distal weakness. See text for abbreviations

Pattern of weakness	Major differential diagnosis
Finger flexors, quadriceps, ankle dorsiflexors	IBM (asymmetric)
	Myotonic dystrophy (symmetric)
Scapulohumeroperoneal	FSHD
Scapular winging	Scapuloperoneal myopathies
Biceps weakness	Pompe disease
Foot drop	LGMD 1B, 2A, or 2I
	Myofibrillar myopathies
	IBM from VCP mutations
Myopathic distal weakness	Distal myopathies
Extrinsic hand muscles weaker than intrinsic hand muscles	
Calf muscles weaker than foot muscles	
Axial weakness (also consider myasthenia gravis	FSHD
and motor neuron disorders)	Polymyositis
Neck extensors (head drop)	IBM
Trunk extensors (camptocormia)	Myotonic dystrophy type 2
	Pompe disease
	Nemaline rod myopathy
	Amyloidosis
Extraocular muscle weakness (also consider	Thyrotoxicosis
myasthenia gravis)	PEO
	OPMD
	Centronuclear myopathy
	Minicore myopathy
Ptosis without extraocular muscle weakness	Myotonic dystrophy type 1
	Congenital myopathies
Early or isolated dysphagia or abnormal speech (also consider	IBM
motor neuron disorders)	Polymyositis
	Myotonic dystrophy
	OPMD
	LGMD 1A

IBM Inclusion body myositis, *FSHD* Facioscapulohumeral dystrophy, *LGMD* limb-girdle muscular dystrophy, *IBM* inclusion body myositis, *PEO* progressive external ophthalmoplegia, *OPMD* oculopharyngeal muscular dystrophy

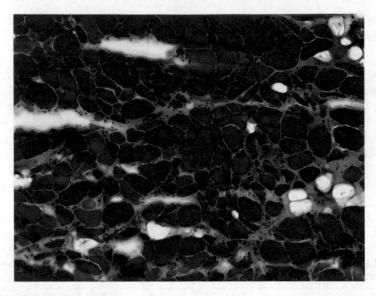

Fig. 2.1 Critical illness myopathy, H&E stain. Note dramatic variation in size and shape of muscle fibers with many atrophic, angular fibers, and pyknotic nuclear clumps

Timing of Symptom Development Is Useful for Differential Diagnosis

Acute (<1 week) myopathic weakness is rare, suggesting rhabdomyolysis or periodic paralysis syndrome. Subacute (weeks to months) weakness suggests immune/inflammatory, toxic, metabolic, or critical illness myopathies (Fig. 2.1). Chronic (months to years) weakness suggests muscular dystrophy, congenital myopathy, metabolic myopathy, or IBM.

Myalgia

Myalgia is *likely* to be due to muscle disease if it is:

- Exercise-induced and not present at rest (as in metabolic myopathies)
- Associated with elevated creatine kinase (CK)
- Associated with examination evidence of myopathy, such as weakness, atrophy, or muscle hypertrophy
- Associated with myopathic findings on EMG

Most cases of myalgia that do not fulfill any of the above criteria are due to non-neuromuscular causes such as fibromyalgia, viral infections, endocrine/metabolic disorders, or polymyalgia rheumatica.

Useful Tests in the Investigation of Myopathies

Serum Creatine Kinase (CK)

- *CK is markedly elevated* (>20× the upper limits of normal) in rhabdomyolysis, toxic myopathies, some muscular dystrophies (Duchenne, Becker, LGMD 2B, 2I, etc.), necrotizing autoimmune myopathies (Fig. 2.2), and anti-synthetase syndrome.
- *CK is moderately elevated* (5–20× the upper limits of normal) in dermatomyositis, polymyositis, several muscular dystrophies, toxic myopathies, hypothyroidism, and Pompe disease.
- *CK is mildly (<3–5×) elevated or normal* in inclusion body myositis, many congenital myopathies, many metabolic myopathies (e.g., mitochondrial, lipid-storage disorders, McArdle), myotonic dystrophy, FSH dystrophy, channelopathies (myotonia and paramyotonia congenita, periodic paralysis syndromes), and in motor neuron disorders such as ALS and Kennedy's disease.
- *Abnormally low CK* is encountered in steroid myopathy, thyrotoxicosis, and malnutrition.

Not every high CK is due to myopathy.   Other common causes include intense exercise, trauma, intramuscular injections/EMG (electromyography), hypothyroidism and renal disease.

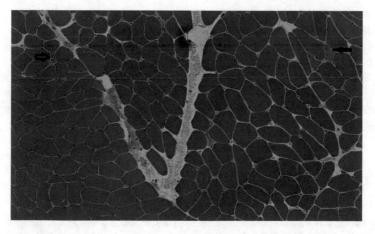

Fig. 2.2 Necrotizing myopathy. H&E stain showing necrotic (left, open arrow) and basophilic, regenerating (right, solid arrow) fibers in the same sample. Also note increased endomysial connective tissue in the fascicles on the right, compared to normal connective tissue on the left, indicating a patchy, multifocal, acquired, as opposed to hereditary, myopathy

Table 2.2 EMG patterns in myopathy and their common differential diagnoses

Spontaneous activity	Voluntary activation	Differential diagnosis
Fibrillation potentials	Myopathic	Inflammatory myopathies Toxic myopathies Rhabdomyolysis Some inherited myopathies

Myotonic discharges	Myopathic	Disorders with clinical myotonia
		  Myotonic dystrophy
		  Non-dystrophic myotonias
		Disorders without clinical myotonia
		  Acid maltase deficiency
		  Centronuclear myopathy
		  Myofibrillar myopathy
		  Hypothyroidism
		  Toxic myopathies
		  Polymyositis

None	Myopathic	Muscular dystrophies Congenital myopathies Metabolic myopathies *Treated* inflammatory myopathies
None	Normal	Steroid myopathy Mitochondrial myopathies Metabolic myopathies

Needle Electromyographic (EMG) Examination

Features of myopathy include abnormal insertional activity (fibrillations, positive sharp waves, and high-frequency discharges, including myotonia) at rest and, during voluntary activity, the presence of small, short-duration, polyphasic motor unit potentials (MUPs) with early recruitment patterns. In some very chronic myopathies (dystrophies, IBM), large, long-duration MUPs can be seen. The differential diagnosis of four specific EMG patterns that can be seen in muscle disorders is listed in Table 2.2. A detailed description of EMG findings is presented in Chap. 8.

Muscle Biopsy

Biopsy of muscle can be performed by open incision or transdermal needle. Part of the muscle sample is rapidly frozen in isopentane cooled in liquid nitrogen. Other parts of the sample can be fixed in formalin, processed for electron microscopy, or submitted for biochemical and genetic testing as needed. Histochemical stains that most laboratories prepare routinely are listed in the table. These can provide extensive diagnostic information. These can be supplemented as needed with electron microscopy, genetic testing, and other immunohistochemical stains to address specific questions (Fig. 2.3).

Stain	Significance	Image
Hematoxylin and eosin (H&E)	Evaluation of structure including fiber shape and size, position of nuclei, presence of inclusions or vacuoles, appearance of blood vessels, state of connective tissue, presence of inflammation, degenerating, necrotic or regenerating fibers	
Gomori trichrome	The same as H&E and presence of ragged-red fibers, nemaline rods, rimmed vacuoles.	
Periodic acid-Schiff	Glycogen content	
Oil Red O	Lipid content in muscle fibers	
Adenine dinucleotide-tetrazolium reductase (NADH)	Mitochondrial distribution, myofibrillar abnormality, fiber types	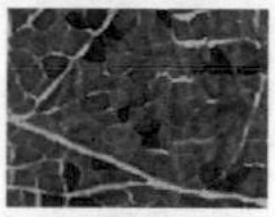
Cytochrome Oxidase (COX)	Mitochondrial presence – reduced activity in fibers devoid of staining	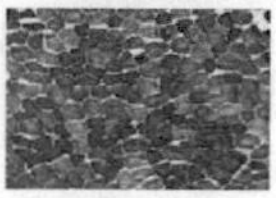
Succinic dehydrogenase (SDH)	Fiber typing and excess of staining (ragged blue fibers) in mitochondrial dysfunction.	
ATPase	Fiber type distribution using ATPases of differing pH.	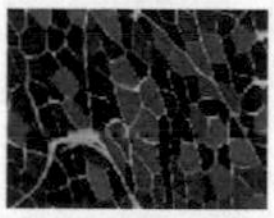
Congo red	Presence of amyloid in muscle fibers and blood vessels	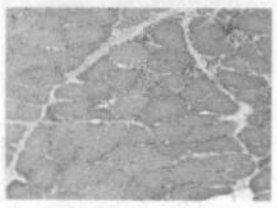
Acid Phosphatase or Fast blue B	Lysosomal activity – high in lysosomal storage disorders, necrotic fibers, and macrophages.	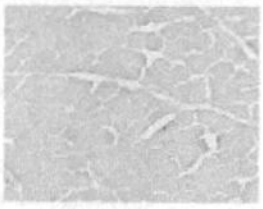

Fig. 2.3 Routine histological and histochemical stains used for evaluation of muscle pathology

While muscle biopsy has been superseded in recent years by genetic testing for certain diagnoses, such as dystrophinopathies, it is still an extremely valuable diagnostic tool when the clinical and electrodiagnostic presentation is nonspecific and in inflammatory myopathies.

Genetic Testing

The rapid expansion of knowledge of genetic causes of muscle disease, coupled with the accelerating reduction in cost of genetic testing, has revolutionized muscle diagnosis. While it remains of critical importance to apply clinical skills in a systematic fashion to develop and refine a differential diagnosis, once one establishes a high pretest probability of a particular genetic diagnosis, the diagnosis can now often be confirmed by identifying the presence of the responsible mutation with genetic testing of leukocytes. Prior to this, many more diagnoses of muscular dystrophy and other genetically determined myopathies required muscle biopsy, which is a moderately invasive procedure. That said, there are numerous pitfalls in genetic testing. Genetic testing is covered in detail in Chap. 10.

Muscle Imaging

Muscle imaging can be done with either MRI or ultrasound. MRI provides considerable anatomic resolution, and contrast enhancement on MRI suggests inflammation in the appropriate clinical context. Ultrasound, by contrast, is less expensive, is not contraindicated by claustrophobia or implanted devices, can be used to evaluate large areas of the body within minutes, and is usually performed by a trained neuromuscular medicine specialist, thus providing the benefit of being an extension of the neuromuscular examination.

Muscle imaging has the following uses:

- Noninvasive assessment of general category of pathology, such as fibrosis, fat infiltration, and edema. Note that imaging cannot, however, confirm inflammation.
- Confirmation of disease-specific patterns of involvement (Fig. 2.4).
- Assistance in guiding choice of muscle for biopsy.

Forearm Exercise Test

The forearm exercise test leverages the fact that glycogenolysis occurs normally with exercise and results in production of lactate. Hence, the absence of a rise in serum lactate after exercise suggests an enzymatic disorder in this pathway.

The forearm exercise test is performed by having a patient squeeze a grip-gauge device or ball at >60% of maximal force repeatedly for 1 minute. The test can be done under ischemic (manometer inflated to above systolic blood pressure) or nonischemic conditions. The ischemic forearm exercise test, however, can cause rhabdomyolysis and compartment syndrome. Blood lactate and ammonia are measured from the non-exercised limb prior to exercise and at regular time points thereafter. Normally, serum lactate and ammonia both rise three- to fivefold after exercise. The lactate peak occurs

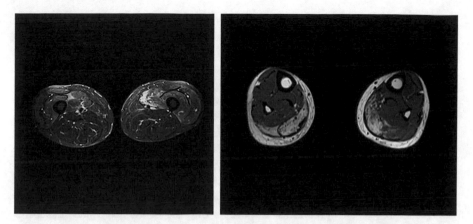

Fig. 2.4 Muscle MRI. Left: Axial T2 images of the thighs in a patient with early inclusion body myositis. Note edema with high T2 signal at the left vastus medialis muscle (right side of image). Also note sparing of hamstring muscles. Right: Axial T1 images of the calves in a patient with Miyoshi myopathy. Note extensive replacement of posterior compartment (gastrocnemius) muscles by fat creating a high T1 signal and sparing of anterior compartment muscles

within 3 minutes, and the ammonia peak occurs within 3 to 5 minutes. Values should return to normal within 40–60 minutes. No rise in lactate with exaggerated rise in ammonia suggests a disorder of glycogen breakdown. No rise in ammonia suggests either poor effort or myoadenylate deaminase deficiency [1].

Case 2.1 illustrates the value of multiple diagnostic tools in establishing a diagnosis in muscle disease.

Case 2.1

A 52-year-old man reported progressive leg weakness over the preceding 10 years. He initially had difficulty getting up from low chairs and ascending stairs. Over the last 2 years, he developed weakness of his shoulder girdle, difficulty lifting his arms overhead, and tripping. He denied dysphagia, dysarthria, ptosis, sialorrhea, diplopia, head drop, or any other symptoms suggestive of cranial nerve involvement. He also denied muscle twitching, bowel or bladder incontinence, dyspnea, orthopnea, non-restorative sleep, morning headaches, or night sweats. He had no difficulty with fine hand movements and denied sensory symptoms. His father died at age 69 and had leg weakness for a number of years prior to his demise. His death resulted from a head injury secondary to a fall from buckling knees. He had three brothers and two sisters, none of whom had been affected by a similar condition. A 75-year-old paternal uncle was wheelchair-bound in a nursing home with dementia and similar weakness, which started in his late 50s. There was no family history of early-onset cardiomyopathy, arrhythmia, or Paget's disease of the bone.

General physical examination was unremarkable. Neurologic examination demonstrated the following: attention, orientation, and recall were normal. Affect and thought content were appropriate. Cranial nerve examination was normal. Neck flexion and extension strength were normal. Sensory examination was normal.

Motor examination demonstrated normal tone throughout but bilateral symmetric scapular winging and atrophy of anterior compartments of the thighs. Manual muscle testing demonstrated bilateral but asymmetric weakness of external rotation at the shoulder (left 4-/5, right 4/5), 4-/5 strength of left elbow flexion, and preserved strength in the distal upper limbs. Hip flexion strength was 3-/5 left and 3/5 right, knee extension strength was 4/5 bilaterally, and distal lower extremity strength was normal. There was abdominal muscle weakness with positive Beevor's sign. Reflexes were trace throughout the upper limbs, absent at the patellae, 2+ at the right Achilles, and trace at the left Achilles. Coordination was normal. He walked with a walker and one-person assist only.

Creatine kinase was elevated at 1800 IU/L (normal <300). Electromyography demonstrated fibrillation potentials and early recruitment of small, short-duration, polyphasic motor unit potentials in multiple muscles of the left upper and lower extremities. MRI of bilateral thighs showed extensive fatty replacement of anterior more than posterior thigh compartment muscles (Fig. 2.5) making quadriceps an unsuitable muscle for biopsy. High-resolution ultrasonography of the left upper extremity showed marked increase of echogenicity with loss of underlying bone acoustic shadow at the left biceps brachii (Fig. 2.6), making it unsuitable for biopsy. Ultrasonography of the left anterior deltoid showed increased echogenicity, with some areas of more normal-appearing muscle, and preserved bone acoustic shadow (Fig. 2.7).

Based on these results, a targeted left anterior deltoid muscle biopsy was performed. This demonstrated evidence of a chronic myopathy, with several fibers demonstrating rimmed vacuoles (Fig. 2.8).

Fig. 2.5 Lower extremity MRI (thighs), T1 without contrast

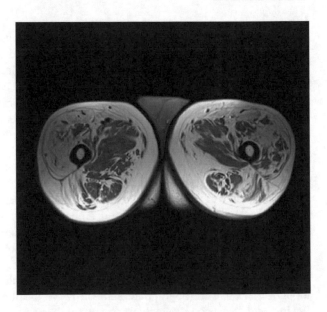

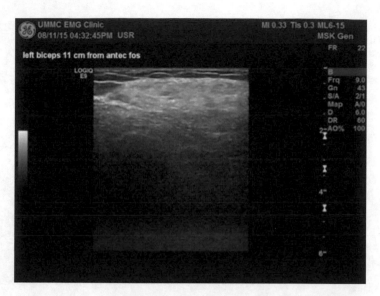

Fig. 2.6 Ultrasonography, left biceps, demonstrating marked increase in echogenicity suggesting advanced muscle fibrosis

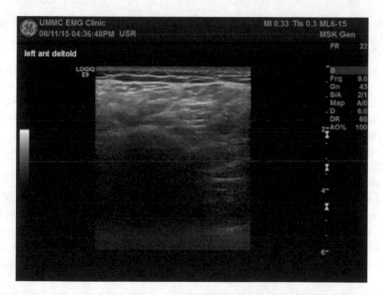

Fig. 2.7 Ultrasonography, left anterior deltoid, demonstrating less severe findings

Based on the autosomal dominant family history of myopathy, the detection of rimmed vacuoles on the biopsy, and the family history of dementia, hereditary inclusion body myopathy with Paget's disease and frontotemporal dementia (HIBM-PFTD [2]) was suspected. Sequencing of the valosin-containing protein (VCP) gene

Fig. 2.8 H&E stain, left
deltoid muscle biopsy,
demonstrating variation in
fiber size, internal nuclei,
and rimmed vacuoles

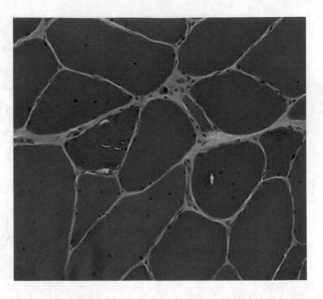

disclosed a variant which was deemed probably pathogenic. The subsequent discovery of another family in which the same variant segregated with the disease phenotype confirmed that it is likely disease-causing.

Discussion: This case demonstrates the role of muscle imaging and genetic analysis in neuromuscular diagnosis. Patterns of muscle atrophy and fatty replacement are, in some cases, nearly pathognomonic and can occasionally obviate the need for biopsy. When muscle biopsy is needed, it is important to choose an area that is affected but not end-stage to maximize yield. As illustrated here, this can be assessed by imaging, but it can also be assessed by manual muscle testing or by NCS/EMG findings.

In this particular case, the diagnosis of inclusion body myopathy was confirmed by muscle biopsy, but the family history indicated that this was more likely a case of hereditary inclusion body myopathy rather than sporadic inclusion body myositis. This was reinforced as well by the presentation more as a limb-girdle phenotype than the characteristic phenotype of sporadic inclusion body myositis, with disproportionate weakness of long finger flexors and quadriceps.

The diagnosis was confirmed by targeted genetic testing of the VCP gene. As discussed in the chapter on genetics of neuromuscular disease, often such testing reveals previously unreported variants of unknown significance. In this case the strong clinical correlation between the phenotype and known VCP mutations and the subsequent description of a family in which this mutation segregates with the phenotype provides supportive evidence of pathogenicity.

Muscle Diseases by Category

Muscle disease is classified into the following categories:

Category	Pathological process
Muscular dystrophy	Mutation of structural protein
Myotonic dystrophy	Repeat expansion mutation
Inflammatory myopathy	Inflammation
Toxic myopathy	Toxic medication, alcohol, other
Metabolic myopathy	Mutation in glycolytic or lipid metabolic pathway
Channelopathy	Mutation in membrane ion channel component
Mitochondrial myopathy	Mutation in mitochondrial or nuclear gene affecting mitochondria
Myopathy due to medical disease	General medical condition affecting muscle
Congenital myopathy	Myopathy presenting in infancy, classified by histopathology

Some muscular dystrophies and congenital myopathies are associated with an increased risk of malignant hyperthermia or rhabdomyolysis after exposure to inhalational anesthetic agents. People with these disorders, as well as individuals with unexplained elevations in serum CK, should be aware of this and be advised to share this information with the anesthesiologist before undergoing general anesthesia.

Muscular Dystrophies

Muscular dystrophies are gradually progressive, inherited disorders leading to muscle fiber necrosis, regeneration, and replacement by connective tissue (fibrosis) or fat.

Duchenne Muscular Dystrophy (DMD)

The most common muscular dystrophy is Duchenne muscular dystrophy (DMD), an X-linked disorder due to dystrophin gene mutations, often large deletions or point mutations leading to stop codons, called nonsense mutations. DMD develops in 1/3500 live male births. Dystrophin anchors the contractile apparatus to the sarcolemmal membrane (Fig. 2.9). The usual age of onset is 3–5 years. Presenting symptoms and signs include proximal (limb-girdle) weakness and calf pseudohypertrophy. Gowers' maneuver is classically present. Affected patients commonly become wheelchair-bound by age 12. Later complications include scoliosis, contractures, respiratory failure, and cardiomyopathy. Screening with an EKG and echocardiogram should start at age 6 and be performed annually after age 10.

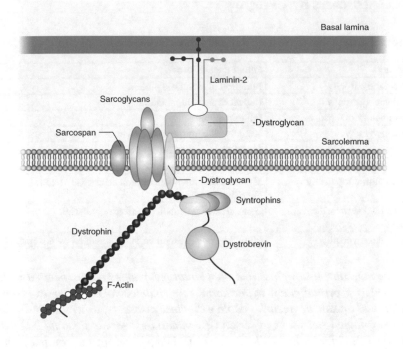

Fig. 2.9 Sarcolemmal membrane and extracellular matrix protein complex. Note that dystrophin anchors contractile elements (F-actin) to the β dystroglycans and sarcoglycan complex

The diagnosis of DMD is confirmed by sequencing of the dystrophin gene. Muscle biopsy provided confirmation of the diagnosis prior to the advent of genetic testing and demonstrates characteristic histologic findings and loss of dystrophin staining. Treatment with steroids (0.75 mg/kg prednisone or 0.9 mg/kg of deflazacort daily) has been shown to delay loss of ambulation by 2–3 years, reduce contractures, and slow rate of loss of respiratory function, at the risk of developing steroid side effects. Recently, an antisense oligonucleotide genetic therapy, eteplirsen, was approved for use in DMD. Eteplirsen produces skipping of exon 51 and restoration of the reading frame, allowing production of a partially functional dystrophin in boys with a deletion in this region, or about 14% of boys with DMD. Other genetic therapies including attempts at delivery of dystrophin gene constructs with adenoviral and other vectors are in development.

Dystrophin mutations also cause a milder phenotype known as Becker muscular dystrophy. Patients with Becker muscular dystrophy are ambulatory until age 16 or much later. The incidence of cardiomyopathy is similar to Duchenne. Most cases of Becker muscular dystrophy are caused by point mutations resulting in alteration of one amino acid without disturbing the reading frame (missense mutations).

Some dystrophin mutations present with yet milder phenotypes, including asymptomatic elevation of serum CK, myalgias, isolated quadriceps atrophy, and cardiomyopathy.

Case 2.2

A 17-year-old boy presented for routine evaluation at the Muscular Dystrophy Association (MDA) care center and consideration for a novel treatment. His initial presentation was at the age of 5 years when he was evaluated by a pediatric neurologist for complaints of abnormal gait, slower running than his peers, and learning difficulties. His parents reported that he was born at term without complication. Perinatal history was uncomplicated as well. Over the course of the first year of life, there were mild concerns regarding his gross motor development because of 1–2 months delay in acquisition of his motor milestones. However, he reached gross motor milestones by the first birthday, such as holding his head up, rolling over, sitting, and standing at normal times. However, he did not walk until the age of 18 months. By the age of 3 years, his parents became more concerned about his development when they noticed a difference in his physical capacity when compared to other boys of his age. Specifically, he was slower than other boys and demonstrated an unusual gait with toe walking. His parents also noticed that his language development was slower, and he did not start to talk until he was 2 years of age. His pediatrician recommended evaluation by a physical therapist.

At the time of his initial evaluation at the age of 5, his physical capacity had improved, but his discrepancy when compared to his peers was becoming more apparent. At that point he was referred to a pediatric neurologist. Clinical evaluation revealed a healthy-appearing well-nourished toddler with appropriate physical development. Neurological examination revealed no abnormalities in his mental status and cranial nerves. Motor examination revealed a Trendelenburg gait and mild hyperlordosis. He had apparent proximal weakness evident by Gowers' sign during standing up from a supine position on the floor. Manual motor examination could not be assessed formally due to inability to cooperate. Calf muscle hypertrophy was apparent (Fig. 2.10). Creatine kinase level was markedly elevated at 24,830. At that point muscle biopsy

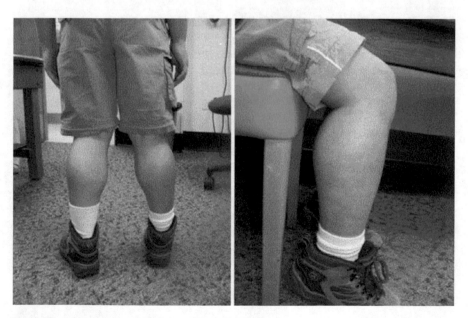

Fig. 2.10 Calf muscle hypertrophy in a boy with DMD

showed findings consistent with muscular dystrophy due to dystrophinopathy. Genetic testing confirmed the diagnosis and found a mutation in the dystrophin gene consisting of deletion of exons 48 through 50. He was started on of 0.75 mg/kg of prednisone.

Over the next several years, he experienced progressive muscle weakness, most notably in the proximal musculature of the arms, pelvis, and legs. He required orthotic braces (nighttime splints) to assist stretching his ankles during sleep. By age 12, he was nonambulatory. In his teens he was still able to use utensils, write, use a keyboard, and drive his wheelchair, though these functions declined over the year prior to his evaluation at age 17, and he now requires full assistance for all activities of daily living.

The patient has no history of muscle pain or spasm, chest pain, or irregular heartbeat. He was diagnosed with a learning disability in elementary school, but has progressed through the grades with an individual educational plan. After loss of ambulation, he discontinued treatment with corticosteroids. He has been followed at the MDA care center at 6-month intervals with close monitoring of his respiratory and cardiac function. He does not have cardiomyopathy at this point. He does have restrictive lung disease with nocturnal hypoventilation, which requires treatment with noninvasive ventilation. While he developed scoliosis, no corrective surgery was required. Recently, he started eteplirsen as a weekly intravenous infusion. The goal is to slow progression of muscle weakness and its complications.

Discussion: This case illustrates a characteristic progression of disease with DMD. Management is complex and requires attention to ventilatory and cardiac function. Steroids have a place in prolonging ambulation.

Facioscapulohumeral Dystrophy (FSHD)

FSHD is an autosomal dominant (AD) muscular dystrophy with an incidence of about 1:20,000 live births, making it the second most common adult onset muscular dystrophy. *Patients with FSHD present with characteristic asymmetric weakness of scapular, humeral (biceps and triceps, with notable sparing of deltoid), peroneal, and facial muscles* (Fig. 2.11). The appearance of the upper body is also characteristic, with asymmetric scapular winging, scapular elevation, and accessory pectoralis folds. Age of onset is variable, from birth to 80 years. Severe congenital forms with sensorineural hearing loss, retinal telangiectasia or detachment (Coats' disease), epilepsy, mental retardation, and respiratory failure have been described. The diagnosis of FSHD is confirmed by genetic testing. In 90–95% of cases, a reduction in the size of a DNA sequence (4q35) in chromosome 4 containing repeat D4Z4 elements is detected. This leads to hypomethylation of DNA and overexpression of a normally silenced downstream gene, DUX4, which may be disease-causing. In the remaining 5–10% of cases, abnormal methylation of the D4Z4 elements, often associated with mutations in the structural maintenance of chromosomes flexible hinge domain containing 1 (SMCHD1) gene is found [3]. Muscle biopsy findings are nonspecific but may show striking lymphocytic inflammation, sometimes leading to misdiagnosis as a primary myositis.

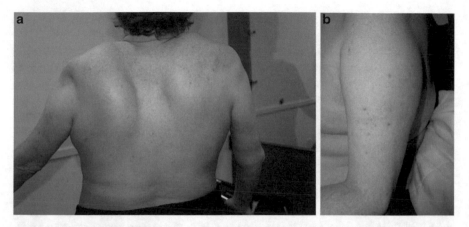

Fig. 2.11 FSHD. (**a**) Asymmetric scapular winging and elevation. (**b**) Atrophy of biceps with relative sparing of deltoid

Myotonic Dystrophy

Myotonic dystrophy is inherited in an autosomal dominant fashion. *Myotonic dystrophy type 1 (DM1) is the most common adult onset muscular dystrophy*. It is caused by a CTG expansion in the DMPK gene, leading to a toxic mRNA product that sequesters RNA-binding proteins, which in turn does not allow proper expression of many mRNAs coding for other proteins [4]. Clinically, it manifests with prominent ptosis, facial weakness, atrophy of masseter and temporalis muscles, frontal balding, distal weakness in handgrip and foot dorsiflexion, and myotonia. *Myotonia is the delayed relaxation of muscle after contraction*, which can be elicited by percussion of the thenar eminence or extensor muscles or by repeated eyelid opening and closing.

DM1 is a multisystem disorder, with the following associated conditions [5]:

- Executive dysfunction and other cognitive disorders
- Cardiac conduction abnormalities
- Ventilatory insufficiency
- Cataracts
- Sleep disorders, including daytime hypersomnia mimicking narcolepsy and central sleep apnea
- Gastrointestinal disorders, such as irritable bowel syndrome
- Endocrine disorders, including diabetes and testicular atrophy
- Cancer, especially skin and thyroid

Heightened awareness and regular screening for these protean manifestations must be part of the care plan for people with DM1. *In particular, an annual electrocardiogram and cardiology evaluation are critical, as sudden death from cardiac conduction abnormalities is the leading cause of death among people with DM1.*

Anticipation, in which subsequent generations have a larger CTG repeat expansion due to instability during meiosis, is a well-recognized phenomenon in DM1. As a result, mildly affected mothers can give birth to infants with severe congenital myotonic dystrophy. Anticipation is discussed in greater detail in Chap. 10.

The diagnosis of DM1 can be suspected on the basis of the clinical presentation and the presence of myotonic discharges in distal muscles on EMG. The diagnosis is readily and reliably confirmed by identification of the repeat expansion on genetic testing. Muscle biopsy shows a large amount of internal nuclei and occasional ring fibers, but those findings are not specific. While there is as yet no specific therapy for DM1, monitoring for and supportive treatment of its multisystem complications as well as the myopathic features is essential. Mexiletine and other sodium-channel blockers can be used for symptomatic myotonia.

Myotonic dystrophy type 2 (DM2, previously called proximal myotonic myopathy, or PROMM) is an AD disorder caused by a CTG expansion in the ZFN9 gene on chromosome 3 [6]. It is common in the upper midwest of the United States among people of Scandinavian and German ethnic origin. Symptoms start later than DM1, often after age 30, and include prominent myalgias and mild-to-moderate limb-girdle, neck flexor, and handgrip weakness. Clinical myotonia is appreciated in less than 50% of patients with DM2. Systemic complications like those in DM1 do occur, and the approach to diagnosis and treatment is similar.

Limb-Girdle Muscular Dystrophy

Limb-girdle muscular dystrophy (LGMD) is a phenotypic classification of a dystrophy with bilateral weakness most prominent in the hip and shoulder girdle regions. LGMD has been associated with numerous mutations in both autosomal dominant (LGMD 1) and recessive (LGMD 2) patterns. The mutations responsible for LGMD are diverse and affect mostly proteins of the sarcolemmal membrane and/or extracellular matrix, but also proteins involved in functions of nuclei, RNA processing, contractile apparatus, and intermediate filaments. The prevalence of individual mutations, particularly LGMD 2 mutations, varies widely based upon ethnicity. Mutations in sarcoglycan genes account for a substantial proportion of childhood-onset recessive forms of LGMD [7].

Distal Myopathies

A number of muscular dystrophies predominantly affect distal muscles, particularly in the lower limb. *Distal myopathies are often differentiated clinically from a length-dependent neuropathy or motor neuron disease by the relative sparing of intrinsic foot muscles despite atrophy of calf muscles.* Many distal myopathies are known by their eponyms, although several responsible gene mutations have been identified. Distal myopathies are generally differentiated between those in which the anterior tibial compartment is more involved and those in which the posterior compartment (gastrocnemius) is more involved (Table 2.3) [8].

Table 2.3 Classification of distal myopathies and some specific causative mutations

Anterior tibial compartment weakness predominates	Posterior tibial compartment weakness predominates
Nonaka myopathy	Miyoshi myopathy
Welander myopathy	Dysferlin mutation
Myofibrillar myopathy due to one of the following mutations:	Anoctamin 5 (ANO5) mutation
Desmin	Centronuclear myopathy from DNM2 mutations
Z-disk associated protein (ZASP)	
Filamin C	
Myotilin	
Udd myopathy	
VCP myopathy	

Oculopharyngeal Muscular Dystrophy

Oculopharyngeal muscular dystrophy (OPMD) is a rare, autosomal dominant, late-onset (often after age 50) muscular dystrophy presenting with slowly progressive ptosis, ophthalmoparesis, and dysphagia. Many, but not all, patients are of French-Canadian origin. The diagnosis is suspected from family history, and confirmed by genetic testing, which demonstrates a trinucleotide repeat expansion in the polyadenylate-binding protein 1 (PABN1) gene in most cases [9]. Muscle biopsy demonstrates rimmed vacuoles, and electron microscopy demonstrates tubulofilamentous nuclear inclusions. Treatment is supportive, including corrective surgery for ptosis and cricopharyngeal myotomy or gastrostomy for progressive dysphagia.

Inflammatory Myopathies

Dermatomyositis

Dermatomyositis (DM) is a relatively common condition. It presents with symmetric limb-girdle weakness, occasional head drop, dysphagia, respiratory failure, and rarely myocarditis (Fig. 2.12). *Dermatologic features include an erythematous scaly rash over the metacarpophalangeal and knee joints and photosensitive rash around the neck. Nail telangiectasias facilitate the diagnosis but are not always present at onset.* Dermatomyositis is associated with connective tissue disorders and malignancy, especially among older patients. *Patients presenting after age 40 must be screened extensively for cancer.* The pediatric form of DM is well-recognized and is a widespread vasculopathy, with skin calcifications and small bowel ischemia, which can be life-threatening. CK in DM is high, typically >3–5 times the upper limit of normal.

The diagnosis of DM is confirmed by muscle biopsy. *The histologic hallmarks of dermatomyositis are (1) perifascicular atrophy, in which groups of atrophic fibers are seen, largely on the periphery of muscle fascicles, presumably due to ischemia;*

Fig. 2.12
Dermatomyositis,
hematoxylin and eosin
(H&E) stain. Note large
perimysial and perivascular
collection of lymphocytes
at top of image. Also note
rather subtle perifascicular
atrophy (arrow) compared
to the more central regions
of the same fascicle

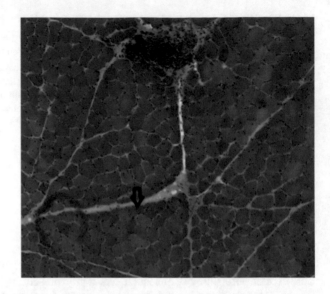

(2) vasculopathy, with loss of muscle capillaries: and (3) perivascular and/or perimysial inflammation, the former consisting mostly of B lymphocytes.

Treatment of malignancy, when identified, is essential and may help stabilize the clinical findings of DM. Regarding direct treatment of DM, however, the first line of treatment is oral corticosteroid therapy. Most patients respond well, but long-term treatment for months or years may be needed, and steroid-related side effects are common. Second-line or steroid-sparing agents such as azathioprine, mycophenolate mofetil, methotrexate, or cyclosporine can be used. Intravenous immunoglobulin (IVIG) or rituximab are third-line treatment reserved for refractory cases.

Case 2.3

A 68-year-old woman developed a sun-sensitive erythematous rash on her face, trunk, and extremities and around her nail beds. A skin biopsy demonstrated features of dermatomyositis. Colonoscopy, mammogram, vaginal ultrasound, and CT of the chest, abdomen, and pelvis were performed and were negative. She was treated with a topical corticosteroid.

About 6 months later, she developed proximal limb weakness and mild myalgias. She had difficulty climbing stairs, standing from a low seat, and holding her grandchildren. Symptoms improved but did not resolve after she discontinued a statin. She was referred for a neuromuscular evaluation.

Neurologic examination demonstrated mild proximal weakness and was otherwise entirely normal. CK and TSH were normal. EMG demonstrated rare fibrillation potentials in thoracic paraspinal muscles only as well as short-duration, low amplitude motor unit potentials and early recruitment in the deltoid muscle. Muscle biopsy demonstrated prominent perivascular and perimysial lymphocytic infiltrates, perifascicular atrophy, degenerating and regenerating muscle cells, and ragged blue or COX-negative fibers, indicative of mitochondrial dysfunction, in a perimysial distribution (Fig. 2.12).

Based upon clinical and pathological criteria, a diagnosis of dermatomyositis was made. Jo-1, SRP, PL-7, PL-12, and Mi-2 antibody studies were all negative. Immunotherapy with prednisone, 40 mg daily, and methotrexate, 5 mg once weekly, was initiated. Her strength and functional capacity gradually returned to normal. Methotrexate dose was titrated upward to 15 mg weekly, and her prednisone dose tapered and discontinued gradually over 3 months' time.

Discussion: This case illustrates several important points about dermatomyositis (DM). First, CK can be normal and weakness relatively subtle despite active disease and clinically meaningful functional disability. Even this patient's EMG was nearly normal, with mild findings restricted to two muscles and fibrillation potentials present in paraspinal muscles only. Nonetheless the muscle biopsy was unequivocally abnormal, with diagnostic features, and the patient demonstrated a good recovery with a tolerable immunotherapy regimen. Before initiating immunotherapy, it is critically important to perform a careful search for occult malignancy in DM, particularly in patients presenting in this age group.

Polymyositis

Polymyositis (PM) is a rare condition and is probably overdiagnosed. The presenting symptoms are similar to those of DM, but a rash does not occur in PM, and PM is very rare in children. As in DM, CK is typically greater than 3–5 times the upper limit of the normal range. PM is frequently associated with connective tissue disorders and less commonly with malignancy (~15–20%). EMG demonstrates fibrillation potentials and a myopathic pattern on voluntary activation. *Because PM is often misdiagnosed in patients with elevated CK and nonspecific symptoms, the diagnosis must be made by muscle biopsy before initiating treatment.* Focal invasion of non-necrotic muscle fibers by lymphocytes, usually CD4+ and CD8+ T cells, and less commonly B cells, is the key feature (Fig. 2.13). Immunotherapy of PM is similar to DM, which is summarized above.

It is important to emphasize that, while both DM and PM result in necrosis and regeneration of muscle fibers, *dermatomyositis is thought to be an inflammatory microvasculopathy, while in polymyositis the primary immune attack is against muscle itself.* Thus, polymyositis is characterized histologically by direct invasion of muscle fibers by lymphocytes, while in dermatomyositis, inflammatory infiltrates are most prominent in the perivascular spaces and perimysial connective tissue.

Anti-synthetase Syndrome

Anti-synthetase syndrome is a distinct form of DM, or less commonly PM, with skin changes (Raynaud's phenomenon, mechanic hands), nonerosive arthropathy, and interstitial lung disease (ILD). Muscle biopsy demonstrates prominent

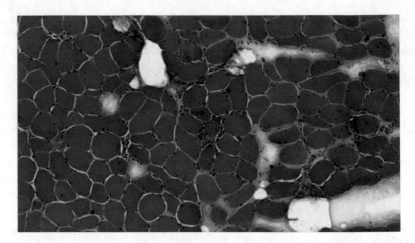

Fig. 2.13 Polymyositis, H&E stain. Note endomysial lymphocytic inflammation with focal invasion of non-necrotic muscle fibers at center and right of image

perimysial fragmentation and macrophage infiltration. It is associated with serum anti-synthetase antibodies, the most common being Jo-1. Patients with this condition must be screened for ILD with pulmonary function studies including diffusion capacity for carbon monoxide (DLCO). Treatment is the same as for PM.

Inclusion Body Myositis

Inclusion body myositis (IBM) is the second most common myopathy in people older than 50 years of age, following statin myopathy [10]. *In most cases the phenotype is so distinctive that clinicians familiar with its appearance can make the diagnosis readily after a brief history and a limited examination of the hands and thighs.* IBM is characterized by asymmetric weakness of long finger flexors, quadriceps, and foot dorsiflexors, with occasional facial weakness as well. The finger flexor weakness can be identified by testing flexion of the distal phalanx in isolation; in IBM it is disproportionately weak, while in most other neuromuscular disorders, it is relatively strong in comparison to intrinsic hand muscles and finger extensor muscles. Patients report difficulty grasping small objects. The quadriceps weakness is also nearly unique to this condition, as this muscle is also relatively spared in other conditions. Quadriceps weakness can be easily overlooked on a casual examination. It becomes most evident when manual muscle testing is done with the knee fully flexed. The typical clinical complaint that results from quadriceps weakness is unanticipated falls, particularly when the knee is not fully extended. Patients will often consciously walk with the knee hyperextended to avoid this.

Dysphagia is present in at least 30% of people with IBM at presentation [11]. In several patients, an abnormal constriction of the cricopharyngeus muscle (sphincter of the upper esophagus) is responsible for the dysphagia.

CK in IBM is mildly elevated or normal. EMG demonstrates fibrillation potentials. While EMG does demonstrate short-duration "myopathic" motor unit potentials, there are also common areas of muscle with reduced recruitment and long-duration, highly polyphasic motor unit potentials and "satellite potentials," or short-duration components appearing well after the main component of the motor unit potential. Hence, EMG in IBM is commonly misinterpreted as neurogenic.

The diagnosis of IBM is confirmed by muscle biopsy, which ideally should show all of the following abnormalities [12] (Fig. 2.14):

1. Lymphocytic inflammation with focal invasion of non-necrotic muscle fibers
2. Rimmed vacuoles
3. Major histocompatibility complex (MHC I) upregulation
4. Aggregates of abnormal proteins, including amyloid, TAR-DNA binding protein 43, p-62, and others

It is not unusual not to appreciate vacuoles or amyloid in the initial biopsy. In those cases, the characteristic pattern of weakness leads to the correct diagnosis.

An antibody against cytosolic nucleotidase 5- 1 alpha (SCN51A) was recently identified in sera of patients suffering from IBM [13]. It is about 50–70% sensitive and 90% specific for the diagnosis. IBM is occasionally misdiagnosed as ALS, likely because it presents as a progressive, painless, pure motor disorder with

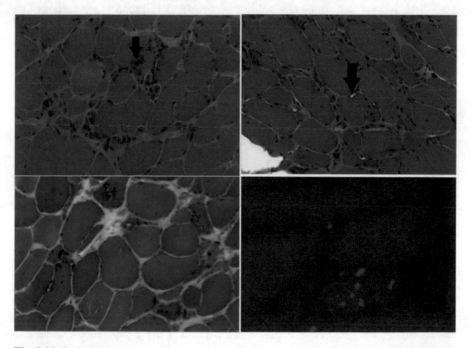

Fig. 2.14 Inclusion body myositis. Upper left: H&E showing focal invasion of non-necrotic fiber by endomysial lymphocytes (arrow). Upper right: H&E showing rimmed vacuoles (arrow). Bottom left: Gomori trichrome showing rimmed vacuoles. Bottom right: Congo red stain visualized under fluorescence microscope showing aggregates of amyloid in muscle fibers

largely preserved reflexes, with a similar age and gender profile, and because the EMG in IBM is sometimes misinterpreted as neurogenic.

The pathophysiology of IBM is currently incompletely understood. The classic pathologic findings suggest both immune and degenerative aspects, and current evidence supports the possible roles of both [14]. Treatment with immunomodulatory therapies has not, to date, provided sustained benefit. IBM is currently a progressive, disabling condition. Although progression is not as rapid as in ALS, IBM can lead to substantial disability. In advanced stages it can lead to loss of ambulation and clinically significant ventilatory dysfunction.

Immune Necrotizing Myopathies

Immune necrotizing myopathies are rare. They cause severe and rapidly (within weeks) progressive limb-girdle weakness, often with respiratory or cardiac involvement. CK is extremely high, more than 20 times the upper limit of normal. The diagnosis is made by muscle biopsy, which shows patchy muscle fiber necrosis but minimal or no endomysial or perivascular inflammation (Fig. 2.2). It is associated with paraneoplastic syndromes, statin exposure with HMG-CoA-reductase antibodies (in contradistinction to the milder toxic myopathy associated with statin exposure discussed below), signal recognition particle (SRP) antibodies, and connective tissue disorders [15]. Treatment often requires high-dose steroids and a second immunosuppressant agent at onset. Occasionally IVIG or rituximab is used in refractory cases. The prognosis is poor unless treated early.

Toxic Myopathies

Statin-Induced Myopathy

Statin-induced myopathy can present in a number of different ways, from asymptomatic hyperCKemia to myalgias with or without CK elevation, to frank rhabdomyolysis. Risk factors for development of statin-induced myopathy include age >70, low weight, female gender, renal failure, diabetes, hypothyroidism, SLCO1B1 polymorphism, and use of other drugs interfering with CYP3A4 [16]. The mechanism of toxicity is uncertain. Interference with CoQ10 and isoprenoid biosynthesis is postulated. The risk of myotoxicity among statins is in this order: simvastatin> atorvastatin> pravastatin> rosuvastatin. Hence, in patients with statin intolerance who have a mild reaction (myalgias, elevated CK) and high cardiovascular risk, rechallenging with low-dose rosuvastatin, such as 5 mg every other day or 2–3 times a week, may be an option.

In patients taking statins who present with abrupt onset of weakness and rhabdomyolysis, it is critical to consider immune-necrotizing myopathy related to statin use with HMG-CoA-reductase antibodies. As noted above, this rare and serious condition requires prompt and aggressive management with immunotherapy and is distinct from the more common toxic myopathy precipitated by statin use. Discontinuation of statin therapy alone is not an adequate treatment of immune necrotizing myopathy related to statin use with HMG-CoA-reductase antibodies.

Colchicine/Amiodarone Toxicity

Colchicine and amiodarone toxicity usually develop in patients with renal failure. These drugs can cause a concomitant myopathy and neuropathy. The neuropathy is demyelinating. Muscle biopsy shows autophagic vacuoles that are acid phosphatase-positive. Nerve biopsy shows characteristic inclusions in Schwann cells.

AZT and Other Nucleoside Reverse Transcriptase Inhibitors

AZT and other nucleoside reverse transcriptase inhibitors are myotoxic. They act by inhibiting mitochondrial DNA polymerase gamma (POLG) [17]. Muscle biopsy shows ragged red fibers on trichrome stain, ragged blue fibers on succinate dehydrogenase (SDH) stain, and cytochrome oxidase (COX)-negative fibers.

Alcohol

Alcohol use can cause a necrotizing myopathy in the context of binge drinking or hypokalemic myopathy.

Corticosteroid Myopathies

Chronic exposure to moderate doses (prednisone over 15–20 mg/day) can cause mild to moderate proximal weakness. CK is low and EMG often normal. Muscle biopsy shows type II fiber atrophy. Acute exposure to high doses of corticosteroids can also cause a more severe condition known as acute quadriplegic myopathy. This condition has several names, including myosin loss or critical illness myopathy, and is discussed in detail below in the section entitled "Myopathies associated with systemic medical conditions."

Both conditions are reversible upon discontinuation of steroids.

Metabolic Myopathies

Metabolic myopathies are genetically determined abnormalities of glycogen and lipid metabolism resulting in impaired energy utilization by muscle. Metabolic pathways of glycolysis and lipid metabolism are demonstrated in Fig. 2.15. The two most common glycogen storage disorders are acid maltase, also known as alpha-glucosidase deficiency (Pompe disease), and myophosphorylase deficiency (McArdle disease).

Pompe Disease

Pompe disease is an autosomal recessive (AR) disorder caused by alpha-glucosidase deficiency and can present in infancy, childhood, or adulthood. *Pompe disease usually produces fixed weakness rather than exercise intolerance. Because the pattern of weakness is limb-girdle, it can mimic any muscular dystrophy or even inflammatory myopathy.* Prominent respiratory failure, occasionally being the presenting feature, is very characteristic. Scapular winging, calf pseudohypertrophy, and tongue weakness are also seen in some patients. Other complications include basilar artery aneurysms and cardiomyopathy. EKG is often abnormal, with evidence of Wolff-Parkinson-White syndrome. CK is usually high, and EMG shows fibrillation potentials and a myopathic pattern on voluntary activation, with myotonic or other high-frequency discharges being especially common in paraspinal muscles. The diagnosis is confirmed by muscle biopsy which demonstrates glycogen accumulation and autophagic vacuoles, which stain with acid phosphatase. Reduced enzyme

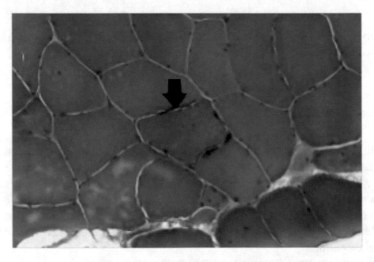

Fig. 2.15 Mitochondrial myopathy. Gomori trichrome stain showing a ragged red fiber (arrow)

activity can also be demonstrated in a dried blood spot. Treatment includes intravenous recombinant alpha-glucosidase, *which can be lifesaving in infants and slows the progression of respiratory failure and weakness in adults.* [18, 19]

McArdle Disease

McArdle disease is autosomal recessive and characterized by exercise intolerance and myalgias with short, intense anaerobic exercise, due to inability to break down glycogen. Rhabdomyolysis can occur and can be life-threatening. *The second-wind phenomenon is characteristic.* This refers to improvement in exercise intolerance and myalgias with brief rest after the first few minutes of exercise and is attributed to utilization of other substrates for energy, such as fatty acids. Mild fixed proximal weakness can occur in later stages. CK and EMG show variable results and are sometimes normal. The diagnosis can be supported by a forearm exercise test showing no rise in lactate and excessive rise in ammonia in the first 3 minutes of exercise. Muscle biopsy with phosphorylase A staining is also diagnostic. Treatment includes sucrose administration before exercise. Some patients may benefit from pyridoxine or ramipril supplementation [20, 21].

Carnitine palmitoyltransferase 2 Deficiency

Carnitine-palmitoyl-transferase 2 (CPT2) deficiency is probably the most common metabolic cause of recurrent rhabdomyolysis in adults. It is autosomal recessive, and manifests with exercise intolerance and myalgias or attacks of severe rhabdomyolysis precipitated by prolonged aerobic exercise. The symptoms arise due to inability of esterified fatty acids to transfer from the cytoplasm into mitochondria. Patients often appear normal between attacks, without weakness. Serum carnitine levels are normal. Raised levels of plasma C16 and C18:1 acylcarnitines can be detected during an episode of rhabdomyolysis or after a 12-hour fast. CK and EMG are normal between attacks, and muscle biopsy usually shows no lipid storage. The diagnosis can be confirmed by genetic testing or by enzymatic analysis of CPT2 activity in muscle biopsy tissue. Supplementing the diet with medium-chain triglycerides or bezafibrate can reduce the frequency of rhabdomyolysis episodes [22].

Channelopathies

Channelopathies are genetic disorders of muscle ion channels resulting in either impaired repolarization, and hence sustained contractions (myotonia), or episodic paralysis because of inability to contract. *All channelopathies except recessive myotonia congenita (Becker disease) are inherited in an autosomal dominant fashion.*

Myotonia Congenita

Myotonia congenita occurs due to chloride channel (CLCN1) mutations [23]. Major symptoms are stiffness and cramps, whereas strength is normal or only mildly reduced. Myotonia improves with exercise and is more prominent in the lower extremities. Muscle hypertrophy is sometimes striking and referred to as a Herculean appearance.

Paramyotonia Congenita and Hyperkalemic Periodic Paralysis

Paramyotonia congenita and hyperkalemic periodic paralysis are related to sodium channel SCN4A mutations [24]. *Paramyotonia refers to paradoxical worsening of myotonia with repetitive exercise.* Onset is earlier than CLCN1 myotonia (1st decade), and eyelid myotonia can be prominent. Paralytic attacks are multiple, generally brief, and triggered by cold exposure, fasting, or stress. Treatment of myotonia includes sodium-channel blockers, such as mexiletine, phenytoin, and carbamazepine, and acetazolamide for periodic paralysis. A clinical diagnosis can be supported by the presence of electrical myotonia on EMG, particularly if performed after cooling the limb, and is confirmed with genetic testing.

Hypokalemic Periodic Paralysis

Hypokalemic periodic paralysis has been identified as a consequence of mutations in the CACN1A calcium channel or, less commonly, the SCN4A potassium channel [25]. There is no clinical or electrical myotonia. Paralytic attacks start in the 2nd to 3rd decade, last up to hours, and can be triggered by heavy carbohydrate load (e.g., a pizza meal), exercise, insulin, or beta-agonists, which trigger an intracellular potassium shift. Weakness is diffuse or focal, but typically spares ocular muscles, and respiratory involvement is infrequent. During a paralytic attack, electrical stimulation of motor nerves yields no response. Hypokalemia is detectable in the early stages of an attack, but rarely between attacks. *Persistent hypokalemia between attacks or onset after age 25–30 suggests a secondary, non-genetic cause of hypokalemia.* Thyroid function should be assessed routinely in adults, as thyrotoxic periodic paralysis can occur, especially in men of Asian origin. The diagnosis is suspected on the basis of clinical and laboratory features and can be confirmed with genetic testing. Between attacks the prolonged exercise test demonstrates a characteristic reduction in CMAP amplitude during repeated muscle contraction. During attacks, treatment consists of potassium supplementation. Between attacks, acetazolamide, dichlorphenamide, or potassium-sparing diuretics are used.

Andersen-Tawil syndrome is due to mutations in the KCNJ2 potassium channel and is characterized by the clinical triad of *periodic paralysis, cardiac arrhythmias (long-QT), and dysmorphic facial features* [26].

Mitochondrial Myopathies

The genetics of mitochondrial disorders is very complex. Mutations of mitochondrial DNA are inherited by maternal transmission. Mutations of nuclear DNA affecting mitochondrial stability or synthesis of certain subunits of the respiratory chain are inherited more commonly in autosomal dominant, and less commonly autosomal recessive, fashion.

Mitochondrial disorders affect multiple organs, including the heart (cardiomyopathy, arrhythmias), endocrine (diabetes, short stature, thyroid dysfunction), retina (pigmentary retinopathy), muscle, peripheral nerve, brain (see below), and liver (Fig. 2.15). The diagnosis of a mitochondrial myopathy can be suspected on the basis of several features including:

- Recognition of a pathognomonic clinical syndrome
- Serum lactic acid, which is often but not always elevated
- Plasma fibroblast growth factor 21 (FGF-21) and growth differentiation factor 15 (GDF-15) levels, which are elevated in about 75–80% of cases
- Aerobic exercise test, such as bicycle ergometry, showing a more than twofold rise in lactic acid after 20 minutes

And confirmed by one of the following:

- Muscle biopsy, showing a significant amount of ragged red, ragged blue, or COX-negative fibers, markedly reduced activity of oxidative phosphorylation enzymes (complexes I–V), or a pathogenic mt-DNA mutation
- Detection of a mt-DNA or nuclear DNA mutation affecting mitochondrial machinery by genetic testing from leukocytes

The following conditions are among the more prevalent and clinically important mitochondrial myopathies.

Kearns-Sayre Syndrome

Kearns-Sayre syndrome (KSS) is identified by the triad of progressive external ophthalmoplegia (PEO), pigmentary retinopathy, and cardiomyopathy (heart block). Onset is typically before age 20. Other common features are ataxia and high CSF protein. PEO can also occur in isolation. Both KSS and PEO in isolation are due to large-scale deletions of mitochondrial DNA, which can be detected only by muscle biopsy and *not* by testing leukocytes.

Mitochondrial Myopathy, Lactic Acidosis, and Stroke-like Episodes

Mitochondrial myopathy, lactic acidosis, and stroke-like episodes (MELAS) usually presents before age 40, with muscle weakness and symptoms of cortical dysfunction including focal neurological deficits mimicking stroke, encephalopathy, and seizures. Brain MRI demonstrates high signal on diffusion imaging; however, unlike stroke, signal intensity is normal on corresponding apparent diffusion coefficient (ADC) images, and the hyperintensities are not restricted to a single vascular territory. Brain MR spectroscopy may show a lactate peak during attacks, and CSF lactic acid is elevated. The diagnosis is made by muscle biopsy and leukocyte genetic testing. A leucine tRNA A3243G mutation is the most common mutation. L-arginine supplementation or corticosteroids can reduce the severity of stroke-like episodes [27, 28].

Myoclonic Epilepsy and Ragged Red Fibers

Myoclonic epilepsy and ragged red fibers (MERFF) is characterized by muscle weakness, myoclonic epilepsy, ataxia, hearing loss, optic atrophy, and dementia. Epilepsy is generalized, photosensitive, and resembles juvenile myoclonic epilepsy. MERRF is diagnosed by muscle biopsy or genetic testing; a lysine tRNA A8344G point mutation is the most common mutation.

Mitochondrial Neurogastrointestinal Encephalomyopathy

Chronic intestinal pseudo-obstruction (recurrent vomiting, cachexia), sensorimotor polyneuropathy (demyelinating, may mimic CMT or CIDP), PEO, and endocrinopathies, sometimes with short stature, are the clinical features of mitochondrial neurogastrointestinal encephalomyopathy (MNGIE). It is usually autosomal recessive due to thymidine phosphorylase mutations. The diagnosis is made by testing serum thymidine and deoxyuridine, which are both elevated in MNGIE. Treatment includes bone marrow transplantation or thymidine-phosphorylase-rich platelet transfusion [29].

Myopathies Associated with Systemic Medical Conditions

Hypothyroidism

Hypothyroidism is a common cause of myalgias, mild proximal weakness, and rarely myoedema (dimple upon percussion of the thenar eminence) and muscle hypertrophy (Hoffman syndrome). Associated features supporting this diagnosis include cold intolerance, myxedema, entrapment neuropathies, and delayed relaxation of Achilles reflexes. CK is usually high. EMG may show fibrillation potentials or myotonia.

Hyperthyroidism

Hyperthyroidism usually produces muscle wasting and atrophy without frank weakness. CK is low. Thyrotoxic ophthalmopathy (Graves' disease) presents with proptosis, optic neuropathy, and a *restrictive ophthalmoparesis*. The most commonly affected muscle is the *medial rectus*, resulting in inability to abduct the affected eye. Forced ductions allow differentiation from paralytic ocular disorders.

Thyrotoxicosis can also cause muscle weakness through its association with myasthenia gravis (exotropia or ptosis should raise suspicion) and with periodic paralysis.

Acute Quadriplegic Myopathy

Acute quadriplegic myopathy (AQM) or "critical illness myopathy" was originally described in patients with severe asthma who were intubated and treated with paralytic agents and high-dose steroids [30], but it can occur in any patient with prolonged ICU stay, regardless of exposure to those medications. Transection of sciatic nerve with simultaneous administration of high doses of steroids reproduces the features of the disease in animal models [31]. Weakness is diffuse (proximal and distal) and may be severe. Inability to wean from mechanical ventilation during recovery from a critical illness is usually the presenting feature. Patients may have a coexisting polyneuropathy, which can cause confusion in interpreting the neuromuscular presentation. CK can be high in the early stages due to muscle necrosis, but at later stages is typically very low. Nerve conduction studies show attenuated, long-duration compound muscle action potentials. EMG often (~60%) shows fibrillation potentials in the earlier stages of the disease due to muscle necrosis. Later, myopathic motor unit potentials are appreciated, without abnormal insertional activity. *If however injury is isolated to myosin filaments and muscle membranes remain intact, fibrillation potentials will not be evident and CK will remain normal or reduced despite severe weakness.* Direct stimulation of muscle endplate may be necessary if the patient is too weak to activate muscles for needle EMG examination [32]. Although this diagnosis is generally made on clinical and electrodiagnostic grounds alone, when a muscle biopsy is performed, it shows selective loss of myosin thick filaments, which is appreciated by ATPase/myosin stains or by electron microscopy. Scattered angular, basophilic fibers with abnormal nuclei are common (Fig. 2.1). Treatment is supportive, and recovery is expected if the patient's medical condition improves, but recovery can be very gradual, taking months or even years before regaining independent function.

Congenital Myopathies

The term *congenital myopathy* applies to a group of static or slowly progressive disorders starting in infancy. They manifest with hypotonia at birth (floppy infant), frequently with respiratory failure. Orthopedic complications, including scoliosis and hip dislocations, are common. CK is often normal, and EMG is inconsistently myopathic. Biopsy is required for specific diagnosis, which is not always possible. Congenital myopathies must be differentiated from other peripheral or central causes of infantile hypotonia, including congenital myasthenic syndromes, spinal muscular atrophy, and congenital muscular dystrophies. Hypotonia in infancy is covered in greater depth in Chap. 6.

The most common congenital myopathy is central core disease due to autosomal dominant ryanodine receptor-1 (RYR1) mutations [33]. Others include nemaline rod myopathies, which are genetically diverse, and centronuclear myopathy, which can be severe in boys with X-linked myotubularin 1 mutations and manifest with ophthalmoplegia and respiratory failure. *Patients with RYR1 mutations are at increased risk for malignant hyperthermia or rhabdomyolysis after exposure to inhalational anesthetic agents. These patients should be advised to share this information with the anesthesiologist before undergoing anesthesia.* Congenital myopathies are also discussed in Chap. 10.

References

1. Tarnopolsky M, Stevens M, MacDonald JR, Rodriguez C, Mahoney D, et al. Diagnostic utility of a modified forearm ischemic exercise test and technical issues relevant to exercise testing. Muscle Nerve. 2003;27:359–66.
2. Kazamel M, Sorenson EJ, McEvoy KM, Jones LK, Leep-Hunderfund AN, et al. Clinical spectrum of valosin containing protein (VCP)-opathy. Muscle Nerve. 2016;54:94–9.
3. Daxinger L, Tapscott SJ, van der Maarel SM. Genetic and epigenetic contributors to FSHD. Curr Opin Genet Dev. 2015;33:56–61.
4. Meola G, Jones K, Wei C, Timchenko LT. Dysfunction of protein homeostasis in myotonic dystrophies. Histol Hitopathol. 2013;28:1089–98.
5. Smith CA, Gutmann L. Myotonic dystrophy type 1 management and therapeutics. Curr Treat Options Neurol. 2016;18:52.
6. Liquori CL, Ricker K, Moseley ML, Jacobsen JF, Kress W, Naylor SL, Day JW, Ranum LP. Myotonic dystrophy type 2 is caused by a CCTG expansion in intron 1 of ZNF9. Science. 2001;293:864–7.
7. Liewluck T, Milone M. Untangling the complexity of limb-girdle muscular dystrophies. Muscle Nerve. 2018.
8. Udd B. Distal myopathies--new genetic entities expand diagnostic challenge. Neuromuscul Disord. 2012;22(1):5–12.
9. Banerjee A, Apponi LH, Pavlath GK, Corbett AH. PABPN1: molecular function and muscle disease. FEBS J. 2013;280:4230–50.
10. Engel WK, Askenas V. Inclusion-body myositis: clinical, diagnostic, and pathologic aspects. Neurology. 2006;66:S20–9.

11. Ko EH, Rubin AD. Dysphagia due to inclusion body myositis: case presentation and review of the literature. Ann Otol Rhinol Laryngol. 2014;123:605–8.
12. Needham M, Mastaglia FL. Inclusion body myositis: current pathogenetic concepts and diagnostic and therapeutic approaches. Lancet Neurol. 2007;6:620–31.
13. Pluk H, van Hoeve BJ, van Dooren SH, Stammen-Vogelzangs J, van der Heijden A, et al. Autoantibodies to cytosolic 5'-nucleotidase 1A in inclusion body myositis. Ann Neurol. 2013;73:397–407.
14. Weihl C, Mammen A. Soradic inculsion body myositis – a myodegenerative disease or an inflammatory myopathy. Neuropath Appl Neurobiol. 2017;43:82–91.
15. Pinal-Fernandez I, Mammen AL. Spectrum of immune-mediated necrotizing myopathies and their treatments. Curr Opin Rheumatol. 2016;28:619–24.
16. Tomaszewski M, Stepien KM, Tomaszewska J, Czuczwar SJ. Statin-induced myopathies. Pharmacol Rep. 2011;63:859–66.
17. Scruggs ER, Dirks Naylor AJ. Mechanisms of zidovudine-induced mitochondrial toxicity and myopathy. Pharmacology. 2008;82:83–8.
18. Kishnani PS, Corzo D, Leslie ND, Gruskin D, van der Ploeg A, et al. Early treatment with alglucosidase alpha prolongs long-term survival of infants with Pompe disease. Pediatr Res. 2009;66:329–35.
19. Schoser B, Stewart A, Kanters S, Hamed A, Jansen J, et al. Survival and long-term outcomes in late-onset Pompe diseae following alglucosidase alpha treatment: a systematic review and meta-analysis. J Neurol. 2017;264:621–30.
20. Sato S, Ohi T, Nishino I, Sugie H. Confirmation of the efficacy of vitamin B6 supplementation for McArdle disease by follow-up muscle biopsy. Muscle Nerve. 2012;45:436–40.
21. Martinuzzi A, Liava A, Trevisi E, Frare M, Tonon C, et al. Randomized, placebo-controlled, double-blind pilot trial of ramipril in McArdle's disease. Muscle Nerve. 2008;37:350–7.
22. Bonnefont JP, Bastin J, Behin A, Djouadi F. Bezafibrate for an inborn mitochondrial beta-oxidation defect. NEJM. 2009;360:838–40.
23. Lossin C, George AL. Myotonia congenita. Adv Genet. 2008;63:25–55.
24. Ptacek LJ, George AL, Barchi RL, et al. Mutations in an S4 segment of the adult skeletal-muscle sodium channel cause paramyotonia congenita. Neurology. 1992;8:891–7.
25. Statland JM, Fontaine B, Hanna MG, Johnson KE, Kissel JT, et al. Review of the diagnosis and treatment of periodic paralysis. Muscle Nerve. 2017.
26. Nguyen HL, Pieper GH, Wilders R. Andersen-Tawil syndrome: clinical and molecular aspects. Int J Cardiol. 2013;170:1–16.
27. El-Hattab AW, Adesina AM, Jones J, Scaglia F. MELAS syndrome: clinical manifestations, pathogenesis, and treatment options. Mol Genet Metab. 2015;116:4–12.
28. Fryer RH, Bain JM, De Vivo DC. Mitochondrial encephalomyopathy lactic acidosis and stroke-like episodes (MELAS): a case report and critical reappraisal of treatment options. Pediatr Neurol. 2016;56:59–61.
29. Lara MC, Valentino ML, Torres-Torronteras J, Hirano M, Marti R. Mitochondrial neurogastrointestinal encephalomyopathy (MNGIE): biochemical features and therapeutic approaches. Biosci Rep. 2007;27:151–63.
30. Hirano M, Ott BR, Raps EC, Minetti C, Lennihan L, et al. Acute quadriplegic myopathy: a complication of treatment with steroids, nondepolarizing blocking agents, or both. Neurology. 1992;42:2082–7.
31. Rouleau G, Karpati G, Carpenter S, et al. Glucocorticoid excess induces preferential depletion of myosin in denervated skeletal muscle fibers. Muscle Nerve. 1987;10:428–38.
32. Rich MM, Bird SJ, Raps EC, McCluskey LF, Teener JW. Direct muscle stimulation in acute quadriplegic myopathy. Muscle Nerve. 1997;20:665–73.
33. Treves S, Jungbluth H, Muntoni F, Zorzato F. Congenital muscle disorders with cores: the ryanodine receptor calcium channel paradigm. Curr Opin Pharmacol. 2008;8:319–26.

Chapter 3
Disorders of Neuromuscular Transmission

Georgios Manousakis

Abbreviations

AchR	Acetylcholine receptor
CMS	Congenital myasthenic syndromes
LEMS	Lambert-eaton myasthenic syndrome
MG	Myasthenia gravis
RNS	Repetitive nerve stimulation
SFEMG	Single fiber EMG
VGCC	Voltage-gated calcium channel

Key Points

- The neuromuscular junction is a specialized structure connecting the presynaptic nerve terminal to the muscle membrane, which utilizes the neurotransmitter acetylcholine.
- Myasthenia gravis (MG) is an autoimmune postsynaptic neuromuscular junction disorder caused by antibodies that either block the acetylcholine receptor or destroy the postsynaptic membrane.
- MG typically presents with fatigable weakness of the ocular and/or bulbar muscles.
- Repetitive nerve stimulation of motor nerves has a sensitivity of ~70–75% for diagnosing generalized MG and <50% for ocular.
- Single-fiber EMG is the most sensitive electrophysiologic technique for the diagnosis of MG, with sensitivity of 98% for generalized disease and >90% for ocular.
- Repetitive nerve stimulation and/or single-fiber EMG may show abnormal results in other neuromuscular conditions, including neurogenic disorders such as ALS.
- Acetylcholine receptor antibodies are detected in approximately 80% of patients with generalized MG and 55% of patients with ocular MG. Of seronegative patients, about 40% have MuSK and 10% LRP-4 antibodies.

G. Manousakis, MD (✉)
University of Minnesota, Department of Neurology, Minneapolis, MN, USA
e-mail: gmanousa@umn.edu

© Springer International Publishing AG, part of Springer Nature 2018
D. Walk (ed.), *Clinical Handbook of Neuromuscular Medicine*,
https://doi.org/10.1007/978-3-319-67116-1_3

45

- Edrophonium (Tensilon) test is utilized infrequently for the diagnosis of MG, due to high frequency of false positive results and cholinergic complications including bradycardia.
- The main symptomatic treatment for MG is pyridostigmine, an inhibitor of acetylcholinesterase that increases the amount of acetylcholine available at the synaptic cleft to bind to receptors.
- Immunomodulatory therapy is required for the majority of patients with generalized MG as well as those with ocular MG who show incomplete symptomatic control with pyridostigmine.
- No immunomodulatory therapy for MG works instantly.
- Prednisone remains the cornerstone of MG immunotherapy. Up to 20% of patients that are treated with high dose (1 mg/kg of prednisone or more) steroids may experience a transient deterioration of their clinical status, which is often preventable by concomitant treatment with IVIg or plasmapheresis.
- Once a satisfactory response to prednisone has been achieved, tapering should be done slowly. Unduly rapid prednisone tapering often leads to relapse of MG.
- Oral immunosuppressants including azathioprine, mycophenolate, cyclosporine, and tacrolimus are used as steroid-sparing agents in MG, but their onset of action is delayed by several months.
- Myasthenic crisis can be precipitated by medical illness, infection, surgery, and certain medications that impair neuromuscular transmission.
- The first priority in the treatment of myasthenic crisis is securing the patient's airway and close monitoring of ventilatory and bulbar function, ideally in an intensive care unit, along with discontinuation of offending agents, treatment of underlying infection, and plasmapheresis or IVIg therapy.
- Thymectomy is beneficial for all MG patients with thymoma, as well as adult patients under the age of 65 without thymoma, with generalized disease, positive acetylcholine receptor antibodies, and disease duration of less than 5 years.
- Lambert-Eaton myasthenic syndrome (LEMS) is an autoimmune presynaptic disorder of the neuromuscular junction, caused by voltage-gated calcium channel antibodies. LEMS is paraneoplastic in about 2/3 of cases and usually associated with small cell lung cancer.
- Unlike MG, LEMS typically presents with fatigable proximal weakness, hyporeflexia, and symptoms of autonomic dysfunction including dry mouth and erectile dysfunction.
- Electrophysiologic studies in LEMS typically demonstrate attenuated CMAP amplitudes and the hallmark finding of CMAP amplitude increment of more than 100% following short isometric exercise of the affected muscle.
- 3,4-Diaminopyridine (3,4-DAP) is a helpful symptomatic treatment for LEMS. History of seizures is a contraindication to its use.
- Botulism is caused by toxins released by *C. botulinum* species which result in impairment of the presynaptic nerve terminal function and decreased release of acetylcholine.
- Unlike GBS, botulism typically presents with descending paralysis, including early ptosis, opthalmoparesis, dysphagia, respiratory failure, and, importantly, autonomic symptoms including constipation and poorly reactive pupils.

- Infantile weakness or hypotonia can be caused by a number of different genetic disorders impacting the function of key proteins of the presynaptic or postsynaptic neuromuscular junction.

Disorders of Neuromuscular Transmission

The neuromuscular junction is a specialized adaptation of the nerve terminal and the muscle cell membrane which allows depolarization of a motor axon to result in depolarization of a muscle cell membrane and, ultimately, contraction of that muscle fiber via excitation-contraction coupling (Fig. 3.1). The motor nerve terminal is a specialized structure containing vesicles of the neurotransmitter acetylcholine. The arrival of an action potential at the presynaptic terminal allows voltage-gated calcium channels in that region to open. The resultant influx of calcium results in the fusion of acetylcholine vesicles with the membrane and release of acetylcholine into the synaptic cleft. The muscle membrane (the postsynaptic membrane) is a highly redundant structure studded with acetylcholine receptors. The redundancy of the postsynaptic membrane and the exceedingly high number of acetylcholine receptors assure effective transmission across the synapse. When a sufficient quantity of acetylcholine binds to the postsynaptic receptors, sodium channels in adjacent muscle membrane open, leading to depolarization of the muscle cell and, in turn, contraction. Disorders of neuromuscular transmission can thus be classified as due to either presynaptic or postsynaptic pathology.

Myasthenia Gravis (MG)

Myasthenia gravis, often referred to as myasthenia, is the most common disorder of neuromuscular transmission and is due to postsynaptic pathology. Myasthenia is caused by antibodies directed against the acetylcholine receptor which either block the receptor site or, more importantly, lead to destruction of the postsynaptic membrane by activation of complement or internalization of receptors. The result is a simplified postsynaptic membrane and enlarged synaptic cleft. This reduces the "safety factor" of neuromuscular transmission and, ultimately, leads to failure of neuromuscular transmission [1].

Myasthenia presents with muscle weakness and fatigue. Fatigue is not only a symptom but can be observed clinically after repeated or sustained muscle contraction. Extraocular and bulbar muscles are usually the most prominently affected, causing ptosis, variable ophthalmoplegia, and weakness of facial, palatal, laryngeal, and pharyngeal muscles. The latter results in dysarthria, dysphonia, dysphagia, and nasal emissions. Asymmetric involvement of cranial muscles is typical. Limb and trunk muscles can be affected, usually in a symmetric fashion. Symptoms are more prominent toward day's end. While myasthenia often begins in the extraocular muscles, the majority (80–90%) of *untreated* patients will develop weakness in other

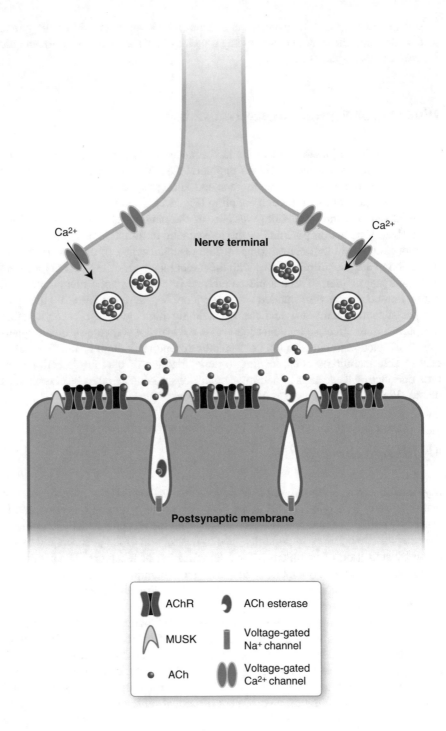

Fig. 3.1 Schematic illustration of the neuromuscular junction

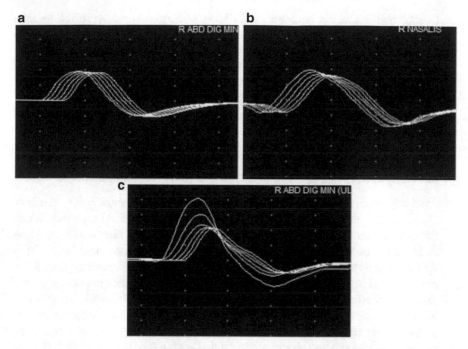

Fig. 3.2 Repetitive nerve stimulation (RNS) at 2 Hz. (**a**) Normal, demonstrating no change in CMAP amplitude with RNS. (**b**) Mild CMAP decrement. (**c**) Severe CMAP decrement

muscles within 2 to 3 years from diagnosis and are classified as *generalized* myasthenia. *Ocular* myasthenia gravis is defined as weakness restricted to the extraocular muscles, which requires a period of observation as noted and eventually applies to no more than 10–20% of patients. In those patients, neurophysiologic testing will often demonstrate subclinical involvement of other muscles. A clinical diagnosis of myasthenia gravis can be confirmed in three ways:

1. Electrophysiologic testing. Repetitive nerve stimulation (RNS) at 2–3 Hz results in a characteristic progressive decrement in the amplitude of the evoked muscle response, as neuromuscular transmission fails in some muscle fibers due to depletion of available acetylcholine (Fig. 3.2). The decrement is generally greatest between the first and fourth stimulus and then improves somewhat, and this typical pattern can be sought when trying to determine whether an apparent decrement is reliable evidence of abnormality or an artifact of limb movement. Sensitivity of this technique for generalized MG is 50% or less when stimulation is limited to distal (e.g., ulnar) nerves and rises to approximately 70–75% with proximal (e.g., spinal accessory, facial) nerve stimulation. However, for purely ocular MG, sensitivity of even proximal RNS is often suboptimal (less than 50%). Maintaining limbs at 32 degrees C or above is of paramount importance, as cooling increases the safety factor for neuromuscular transmission and may result in a false-negative study.

In single-fiber electromyography (SFEMG), abnormal variation in the relative latency of muscle fiber contraction can be demonstrated when two fibers innervated by the same motor neuron are compared. This abnormal variation, called "jitter," is also an indication of impaired neuromuscular transmission. Sensitivity of this technique is much higher than RNS and estimated at 90–95% for ocular MG and 98% for generalized MG [2].

Neither RNS nor SFEMG abnormalities are specific to the diagnosis of MG. Any condition creating immature neuromuscular junctions, including early reinnervation of the muscle after denervation in ALS, can produce similar results. Decrement on RNS can also occur in myotonic disorders and metabolic myopathies. Hence, the results of RNS and SFEMG must be interpreted in the clinical context.

2. Antibody testing. Serum antibodies that bind to the acetylcholine receptor (AchR) are present in at least 80% of people with generalized myasthenia and 55% of people with purely ocular myasthenia. Among patients with negative AchR-antibody testing ("seronegative myasthenia"), 38% have positive antibodies to muscle-specific kinase (MuSK), and another 10% test positive for LRP-4 antibodies. Both antibodies target proteins that form a complex necessary for the proper clustering of acetylcholine receptors at the postsynaptic membrane. MuSK-positive patients have a more aggressive form of myasthenia that is characterized by atrophy of facial and tongue muscles, frequent respiratory muscle involvement and abrupt clinical deterioration ("myasthenic crisis"), poor response or worsening of symptoms with pyridostigmine, no thymic pathology, and dependence on immunotherapy to maintain remission.

3. Rapid improvement of ptosis or limb weakness after administration of anticholinesterase medications, such as intravenous edrophonium (Tensilon®), which enhances the availability of acetylcholine at the synapse. This test is used infrequently as it is prone to false positive results as well as cholinergic complications such as nausea, vomiting, and bradyarhythmia.

Management of myasthenia includes both *symptomatic* and *immunomodulatory* treatments. Symptomatic treatment includes oral pyridostigmine (Mestinon®), which inhibits acetylcholine reuptake, thus increasing the availability of the neurotransmitter in the neuromuscular junction and increasing the likelihood of effective neuromuscular transmission. Pyridostigmine is available in immediate and extended release forms. It is typically started at 30–60 mg every 4–6 hours, and effects are appreciated within 1–2 hours. Adverse effects are mostly cholinergic gastrointestinal symptoms such as cramps, diarrhea, and nausea, which can be alleviated with antispasmodics if necessary. Pyridostigmine alone may be sufficient for patients with mild ocular myasthenia. Very high doses (over 600 mg daily) can produce "cholinergic crisis," manifesting with excess secretions and worsening weakness. This is rare.

Immunomodulatory treatment is required for the majority of individuals with generalized MG and those with ocular MG who continue to have inadequately controlled ptosis or diplopia on pyridostigmine. *It is important to know that no immunomodulatory therapy for myasthenia works instantly.* Intravenous immunoglobulin (IVIg) or plasmapheresis (PLEX) produces a maximum benefit after an average of 5–10 days, corticosteroids such as prednisone after 2–4 weeks, and oral immunosuppressants including azathioprine, mycophenolate, cyclosporine, or tacrolimus, after 3–6 months or more. *Therefore, the choice of therapy largely depends on the urgency of the situation.* For outpatients with moderate, non-life-threatening myasthenic weakness, prednisone is the mainstay of therapy. Prednisone can be started at high doses of 1 mg/kg/day or more and is almost universally effective. *About 20% of patients placed on high-dose prednisone will experience substantial transient worsening of their weakness after 1–2 weeks, sometimes necessitating hospital admission. Hence, if this approach is chosen, patients require close follow-up, and consideration should be given to a course of IVIg or PLEX at the same time.* Alternatively, prednisone can be started at 5–10 mg daily and increased in 5 mg increments weekly, which prevents the phenomenon of clinical deterioration attributed to steroids. This approach is used in patients with milder myasthenic weakness, because it may take more than 4–6 weeks to appreciate the full effect. Once a sustained response is achieved, prednisone is tapered very gradually, generally over a period of months to years. *Unduly rapid tapering commonly leads to relapse, particularly when the dose drops below 20–30 mg/day.* Oral immunosuppressants are often used as adjuncts to allow a more rapid steroid taper and are occasionally used alone in patients who are considered high risk for chronic steroid use. As noted above, however, the effect of "steroid-sparing" immunosuppressants such as azathioprine, mycophenolate mofetil, cyclosporine, or tacrolimus is delayed by several months, so using them alone is often not feasible. If steroids are contraindicated, IVIg can be used to effect a more rapid clinical response and then tapered, with clinical monitoring, 3–6 months after starting oral immunosuppressant therapy. For very refractory patients with MG, newer monoclonal antibodies targeting B-cell precursors (rituximab), or complement activation (eculizumab), appear promising.

Myasthenic crisis is the rapid clinical deterioration of a patient with myasthenia, leading to life-threatening dysphagia or ventilatory failure. It can occur spontaneously, following a medical illness (commonly infection), or due to exposure to drugs that worsen neuromuscular transmission (including but not limited to macrolide, aminoglycoside, or fluoroquinolone antibiotics, muscle relaxants or paralytics, or certain anti-arrhythmic drugs). *Myasthenic crisis can be life-threatening and should be managed with hospital admission to an intensive care unit if necessary, with close monitoring of bulbar and ventilatory function.* Management of ventilatory failure in myasthenic crisis is discussed in detail in Chap. 9. PLEX and IVIg are used in myasthenic crisis because they lead to clinical improvement much faster than all other immunomodulatory treatments. Chronic IVIg or PLEX therapy is generally not preferred and reserved for individuals who do not respond to other medications.

Thymectomy is also commonly used as a treatment in myasthenia gravis. Both B- and CD4+ T-cells that recognize the acetylcholine receptor have been found in the thymus in myasthenia gravis. Thymectomy was recently demonstrated in a randomized single-blinded trial to benefit adults under the age of 65 with generalized AchR antibody-positive MG when performed within 5 years from symptom onset [3]. It appears to be less effective in older patients, and its use in patients with ocular myasthenia is controversial. About 10% of patients with myasthenia have a thymoma, a tumor of the thymus gland, that is usually, but not always, histologically benign. Thymectomy is recommended in all patients with thymoma.

Case 3.1

A 61-year-old man with a past medical history of hypertension and diabetes, on oral metformin, presented with a 1-month history of ptosis and diplopia. He noticed it after a hot shower. Initially the ptosis was noted on the right; subsequently, similar but milder symptoms affected the left eyelid. He endorsed worsening of his ptosis with prolonged reading, and the problem was typically worst in the evening. His diplopia was variable, occasionally horizontal but at other times vertical. Diplopia disappeared when covering either eye. He saw an optometrist for this problem, who prescribed a prism lens on his eyeglasses, which did not help. He was evaluated by another neurologist who ordered an MRI of the brain and orbits with contrast, which showed no pathology in the orbits, cavernous sinuses, or brain stem.

Examination showed variable eyelid ptosis, greater on the right, which worsened upon sustained upward gaze for 1 minute. Manual elevation of the ptotic right eyelid resulted in worsening of ptosis on the left ("curtain sign"). After 10 seconds of sustained downward gaze, the patient's gaze was redirected to the midline, and a transient overshoot of the right eyelid ("Cogan's lid twitch") was detected. Application of an ice pack to the orbit for 1 minute led to reversal of the right ptosis. There was a right eye mild exotropia, discovered upon cover/uncover testing, and a left eye hypertropia. There was moderate weakness of orbicularis oculi bilaterally. Pupillary reactions to light and accommodation were normal. There was no weakness of orbicularis oris, pterygoids, genioglossus, or palatal muscles. There was no dysarthria and no facial or tongue fasciculations. Strength of neck flexion, neck extension, and all limb muscles was normal, without objective fatigue after sustained contraction. Sensation, reflexes, coordination, and gait were normal.

Acetylcholine receptor binding antibody level was elevated (40 nMol/L, normal <0.8). Computed tomography of the chest showed no evidence of thymic tumor or hyperplasia.

Based on serological studies and clinical presentation, he was offered treatment for ocular myasthenia gravis without electrophysiological studies. Pyridostigmine at 60 mg four times a day produced a modest improvement but not complete resolution of his symptoms, with ptosis and diplopia still occurring in the evening and interfering with his activities of daily living, including reading and driving. He also experienced mild diarrhea and abdominal cramping from pyridostigmine. Subsequently, and following consultation with patient's primary care provider, alternate-day oral prednisone was offered, starting at 20 mg every other day, and was gradually escalated to 40 mg every other day. Peptic ulcer prophylaxis was prescribed. The patient experienced insomnia and mild weight gain on prednisone. He had to use short-acting insulin and increase his metformin dose to keep his diabetes under control.

Two months later, his neurological examination had markedly improved, with minimal residual ptosis, normal ocular alignment, and no diplopia. He was able to read at night and to drive. Prednisone dose was gradually tapered over a 4–5-month period to 10 mg every other day, without recurrence of symptoms.

One year after onset of symptoms, the patient experienced an upper respiratory infection. His primary care provider prescribed azithromycin 500 mg twice a day. Because the patient was experiencing cramps on pyridostigmine, he also began self-medicating with high doses of oral magnesium (as much as 1000 mg daily). He then developed recurrence of ptosis and diplopia as well as dysphagia and labored breathing. Examination in the emergency department at that time demonstrated a low-grade fever, tachypnea, and use of accessory muscles of breathing. Cranial nerve examination demonstrated bilateral severe ptosis, severe weakness of extra-ocular muscles, and weakness of orbicularis oculi, orbicularis oris, genioglossus, and neck flexion. Manual muscle testing of the limbs demonstrated moderately severe weakness of shoulder abduction and elbow extension and full strength elsewhere. Forced vital capacity was 1.2 liters, which was 27% of the predicted value. Maximal inspiratory pressure was -20 cm H_2O.

He was diagnosed with myasthenic crisis, likely precipitated by respiratory infection, macrolide antibiotics, and magnesium. The above medications were discontinued. He was electively intubated due to worsening respiratory distress. Pyridostigmine was stopped due to a concern that it would increase secretions. A nasogastric tube and a double-lumen subclavian catheter were inserted, and PLEX, every other day for five sessions, was administered. Blood and respiratory cultures were obtained, and beta-lactam broad-spectrum antibiotics were given. The prednisone dose was gradually increased every 3–5 days to 40 mg daily. Because of his history of diabetes, and in order to facilitate corticosteroid taper in the future, azathioprine was started after the patient's fever resolved and his respiratory infection appeared to be improving. He gradually improved and was extubated and discharged to an acute rehabilitation unit.

At a follow-up visit 4 weeks later, he was breathing independently and had full strength in the limbs. Dysphagia and dysarthria had resolved, but he still demonstrated modest right ptosis and minimal diplopia.

Discussion: This case illustrates several important issues in myasthenia gravis management:

- MG can present as a purely ocular phenomenon and later progress to generalized MG. If it remains purely ocular for more than two years it is likely to remain ocular only.
- The case illustrates several features on examination that can facilitate the diagnosis, including improvement with cooling, which improves the safety factor for neuromuscular transmission.
- Myasthenic crisis is a life-threatening emergency and can be precipitated by systemic infection, rapid steroid tapering, and certain medications. People living with MG should be aware of medications that can exacerbate the condition; a brief list of such drugs is available on the website of the Myasthenia Gravis Foundation of America (myasthenia.org).
- People with ventilatory impairment from myasthenic crisis should all be hospitalized. Because people in myasthenic crisis often worsen continuously until days after treatment is initiated, monitoring in an intensive care unit and elective intubation should be strongly considered if their trajectory suggests that ventilatory failure is imminent, rather than waiting until it is emergent. This is addressed in greater detail in Chap. 9.
- PLEX and IVIg are both beneficial in improving symptoms of MG quickly, often within days, and therefore either one is a mainstay of therapy for myasthenic

crisis. Once again, however, as even these do not provide immediate benefit, stabilizing the patient's medical condition, with mechanical ventilation if necessary, is paramount.

- Steroid therapy is very effective in MG but generally does not take effect for a minimum of 2–3 weeks.
- "Steroid-sparing agents" such as azathioprine and mycophenolate mofetil help enable steroid tapering in patients with MG who are at high risk for serious adverse effects of steroid therapy; however, they do not demonstrate a benefit until 3–6 months after initiation.

Lambert-Eaton Myasthenic Syndrome (LEMS)

Lambert-Eaton Myasthenic Syndrome (LEMS) is a rare acquired presynaptic disorder of neuromuscular transmission. LEMS is caused by an antibody to the voltage-gated calcium channel (VGCC) and can occur either in isolation or as a paraneoplastic syndrome, most commonly in association with small cell lung carcinoma. Detection of serum SOX-1 antibodies increases the likelihood that LEMS is paraneoplastic [4]. Symptoms of LEMS often develop before the tumor becomes symptomatic, which may reflect a beneficial effect of the immune response in suppressing tumor growth. As indicated above, release of acetylcholine from the nerve terminal is triggered by calcium influx via VGCCs. Thus, blockade of VGCCs leads to impaired acetylcholine release and, in turn, impaired neuromuscular transmission.

The clinical presentation in LEMS differs from that seen in myasthenia. In LEMS, patients typically present with mild to moderate bilateral proximal weakness with hypo- or areflexia. Ptosis and opthalmoparesis can be seen, but they occur much less commonly than in MG. LEMS is also associated with autonomic findings such as anhidrosis, dry mouth, and erectile dysfunction.

Antibodies to VGCCs are detectable in the serum in most patients with LEMS. Neurophysiologic studies show characteristic abnormalities. As in myasthenia, 2–3 Hz repetitive nerve stimulation often demonstrates a decremental response. In LEMS, however, routine motor nerve conduction studies demonstrate a low amplitude response in most if not all muscles. After rapid repetitive stimulation or a sustained voluntary contraction, there is a transient but marked increment in the amplitude of the response (Fig. 3.3). This is not common in myasthenia unless the deficit is very severe. The increment after exercise in LEMS occurs because sustained or repetitive contraction facilitates calcium entry through available VGCCs, thus enhancing the chance of effective acetylcholine release after the subsequent test stimulus.

Treatment of LEMS is generally less satisfactory than treatment of myasthenia. Perhaps the most important initial intervention is an aggressive search for malignancy, including computerized tomography (CT) and/or positron emission tomography (PET) scans. Treatment of a tumor, when one is found, may result in improvement in neurologic symptoms. LEMS can be treated with symptomatic therapy as well as

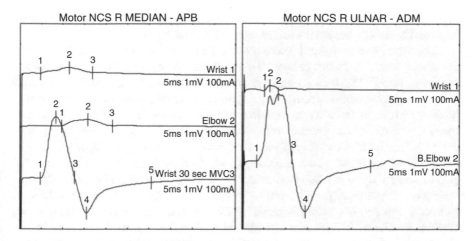

Fig. 3.3 CMAP increment in LEMS. The top two traces on the left and the top trace on the right are CMAPs obtained in a routine nerve conduction study in a patient with LEMS. The bottom traces in both examples demonstrate a marked increment in CMAP amplitude obtained after 30 seconds of maximal voluntary contraction

immunotherapy. Pyridostigmine produces transient and typically incomplete relief. 3,4-Diaminopyridine (3,4-DAP) is a very efficient treatment which blocks the potassium channel responsible for restoring the resting membrane potential after nerve depolarization. This results in prolonged depolarization of the nerve terminal and, in turn, prolonged opening of the voltage-gated calcium channel. 3,4-DAP is not FDA approved and is contraindicated in patients with a history of seizures. Paresthesias are a common side effect.

Immunotherapy is necessary in a number of patients with LEMS. Steroids, azathioprine, PLEX, and IVIg have all been used, with less consistent benefit than in myasthenia. Because the pathogenic antibodies may suppress tumor growth, azathioprine or other immunosuppressant treatments are best avoided until appropriate investigations for malignancy are completed and, if found, treatment of tumor is completed as well. The likelihood of LEMS being paraneoplastic and the necessity of repeat imaging to search for malignancy can be predicted by recently developed algorithms [4].

Botulism

Botulism is caused by toxins (most commonly A, B, and rarely E or other strains) released from *Clostridium botulinum*, a ubiquitous anaerobic pathogen present in soil. The most common form of botulism in the United States is infantile botulism, which has been linked to honey-containing formulas. The toxin is generated in vivo by *Clostridia* which survives in the small intestine of the infant because their bacterial flora is immature and cannot eradicate them. Clinical signs develop when the toxin enters the bloodstream. Less common, but more morbid, forms are food-borne or wound botulism, the latter usually seen in intravenous drug users.

Botulinum toxins inhibit proteins necessary for fusion of acetylcholine-containing vesicles to the presynaptic membrane or exocytosis of the vesicles, including SNAP-25 (toxin A) and synaptobrevin (toxin B). The result is reduced release of acetylcholine from the presynaptic terminal into the synaptic cleft, leading in turn to inability to generate end-plate potentials at the postsynaptic membrane and neuromuscular transmission failure. Because the toxin inhibits acetylcholine release in presynaptic autonomic and enteric ganglia, initial manifestations of botulism often include constipation and poorly reactive, dilated pupils. The paralysis is often descending, in contrast to Guillain-Barre syndrome, with ptosis, ophthalmoparesis, and dysphagia occurring first. Ventilatory failure can occur rapidly. Diagnosis is made by electrophysiologic studies, which show findings similar to LEMS. Identification of *C. botulinum* toxin by PCR or isolation of the pathogen from stool, GI aspirate, or wound culture is generally a less sensitive and more time-consuming approach. Treatment is symptomatic and intubation is often necessary. A fully humanized antitoxin is available for infants less than 1 year of age. In adults, equine antitoxin is used, which can produce serum sickness syndrome [5].

Congenital Myasthenic Syndromes (CMS)

Several mutations in genes coding for both pre- and postsynaptic components of the neuromuscular junction have been described [6]. These present clinically with hypotonia and weakness in cranial and limb muscles in infancy, childhood, or rarely adulthood. The differential diagnoses include a broad range of neuromuscular conditions, but congenital myasthenic syndrome (CMS) should be considered when infants or children present with weakness without sensory deficits. These conditions are discussed further in the chapter on the hypotonic infant.

References

1. Vincent A, Palace J, Hilton-Jones D. Myasthenia gravis. Lancet. 2001;3572:122–8.
2. Howard JF Jr. Electrodiagnosis of disorders of neuromuscular transmission. Phys Med Rehabil Clin N Am. 2013;24:169–92.
3. Wolfe GI, Kaminski HJ, Aban IB, et al. Randomized Trial of Thymectomy in Myasthenia Gravis. N Engl J Med. 2016;375:511–22.
4. Titulaer M, Maddison P, Sont J, et al. Clinical Dutch-English Lambert-Eaton Myasthenic Syndrome (LEMS) tumor association prediction score accurately predicts small-cell lung cancer in the LEMS. J Clin Oncol. 2011;29:902–8.
5. Cherington M. Botulism: update and review. Seminars in neurology. 2004;24:155–63.
6. Souza P, Batistella G, Lino V, et al. Clinical and genetic basis of congenital myasthenic syndromes. Arq Neuropsyquiatr. 2016;74:750–60.

Chapter 4
Motor Neuron Disorders

David Walk

Abbreviations

ALS	Amyotrophic lateral sclerosis
EMG	Electromyography
FTD	Frontotemporal dementia
FUS	Fused in sarcoma protein
IBM	Inclusion body myositis
MRI	Magnetic resonance imaging
MMN	Multifocal motor neuropathy
NCS	Nerve conduction studies
PLS	Primary lateral sclerosis
SBMA	Spinobulbar muscular atrophy
SMA	Spinal muscular atrophy
SOD1	Superoxide dismutase

Key Points
- The diagnosis of ALS is based upon the presence of both upper motor neuron signs, such as hyperreflexia or spasticity, and lower motor neuron signs, such as atrophy or weakness, with progression of disease and adequate exclusion of other conditions that might present in this fashion.

  - While 90% of people with ALS have no family history of the disease, the C9orf72 repeat expansion is found in at least 50% of people with known familial ALS and at least 5% of people with no family history of ALS. The C9orf72 repeat expansion can cause both ALS and frontotemporal dementia (FTD).
  - Both riluzole and noninvasive ventilation (NIV) have been shown to prolong survival in ALS. Edaravone has been approved by the US FDA as a treatment to slow progression of functional deficits in ALS.

D. Walk, MD (✉)
University of Minnesota, Department of Neurology, Minneapolis, MN, USA
e-mail: walkx001@umn.edu

© Springer International Publishing AG, part of Springer Nature 2018
D. Walk (ed.), *Clinical Handbook of Neuromuscular Medicine*,
https://doi.org/10.1007/978-3-319-67116-1_4

- – Management of ALS is complex and should address the following: ventilatory dysfunction, weight maintenance, safe swallowing and timing of gastrostomy, communication barriers, management of sialorrhea, falls prevention, assistance in ADLs, mobility aids, advance care planning including advanced directive, and assessment of mood, pseudobulbar affect, cognitive, and behavioral problems.
- • Primary lateral sclerosis (PLS) is a sporadic motor neuron disorder presenting with progressive upper motor neuron dysfunction. The cause is unknown. The condition can progress to ALS but generally does not if it has not done so for 3–5 years after onset.
- • SMA is a fatal autosomal recessive disorder caused by a deletion or mutation of the SMN1 gene. It presents with progressive proximal weakness in newborns, infants, or children. SMA is now treatable with nusinersen, an antisense oligonucleotide that allows increased production of a functional gene product. Other treatments are in development.
- • SBMA is an X-linked disroder caused by a repeat expansion in the androgen receptor gene and presenting with prominent bulbar and limb muscle weakness, mild sensory neuropathy, and androgen insensitivity in males.
- • Poliomyelitis is due to selective injury to motor neurons of the anterior horn and brainstem from infection with poliovirus or other enteroviruses.
- • Hirayama disease is a condition, typically presenting in adolescent or young adult men, characterized by progressive unilateral or bilateral weakness and atrophy of intrinsic and extrinsic hand muscles.

  - – Hirayama disease has been postulated to be caused by recurrent vascular compromise to the anterior horn due to anterior compression of the cord in individuals with a developmentally taut posterior dura during neck flexion.

Introduction

Voluntary muscle is innervated by motor neurons in the brainstem nuclei and the anterior horn of the spinal cord. These neurons are in turn innervated by cortical motor neurons of the primary motor cortex (Fig. 4.1). While motor neurons can be damaged in a wide variety of pathologic processes, several disorders selectively target motor neurons. These include amyotrophic lateral sclerosis, primary lateral sclerosis, spinal muscular atrophy, focal motor neuron disease, X-linked spinobulbar muscular atrophy (or Kennedy's disease), and poliomyelitis.

Amyotrophic Lateral Sclerosis

Diagnosis of ALS

ALS is characterized by gradual, progressive loss of both cortical ("upper") as well as bulbar and spinal ("lower") motor neurons. It is this combination of upper and lower motor neuron disease that makes ALS unique. Clinically, this is revealed by the

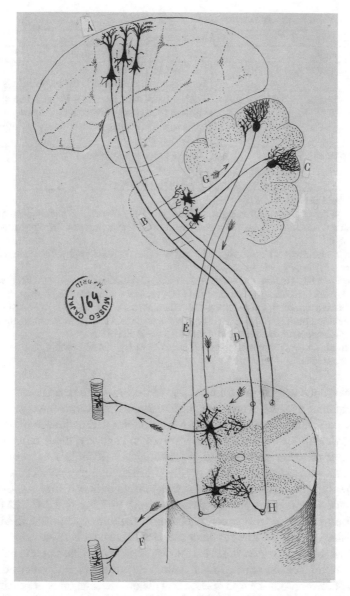

Fig. 4.1 Upper and lower motor neurons drawn by Ramon y Cajal. Note upper motor neuron axons descending via lateral corticospinal tract to synapse with lower motor neurons and lower motor neuron axons exiting the spinal cord to synapse at neuromuscular junctions. Cajal noted the presence of both crossed and uncrossed corticospinal tract fibers, as well as synapses with cerebellar Purkinje cells (Courtesy of Instituto Cajal)

presence of hyperreflexia, pathologic reflexes, or spasticity, all signs of upper motor neuron disease, combined with muscle atrophy and weakness – signs of lower motor neuron disease – in the absence of sensory, cerebellar, or extrapyramidal symptoms or signs. Fasciculations, which can be seen in a variety of disorders of anterior horn

Table 4.1 Revised El Escorial criteria for the diagnosis of ALS

El Escorial classification	Required features
Clinically definite ALS	UMN + LMN in three regions
Clinically probable ALS	UMN + LMN in three regions Some UMN findings rostral to LMN findings
Clinically probable ALS – laboratory supported	UMN + LMN in one region + EMG in two regions OR UMN in one region + EMG in two regions AND appropriate imaging/laboratory exclusion of other potential causes
Clinically possible ALS	UMN + LMN in one region OR UMN in two regions

Abstracted from Brooks et al. [1]

UMN refers to upper motor neuron signs, defined generally as spasticity, pathologic hyperreflexia, or preserved reflexes in weak, wasted myotomes. The criteria accept pseudobulbar affect as a cranial UMN sign

LMN refers to lower motor neuron signs, defined as weakness and atrophy. There are four *regions*: cranial, cervical, thoracic, and lumbosacral

EMG refers to EMG findings of active denervation (fibrillations or positive sharp waves) and chronic denervation (reduced recruitment and large motor unit potentials) in one muscle in the cranial or thoracic region or two muscles with different nerve and root innervation in the cervical or lumbosacral region. The Awaji criteria for the diagnosis of ALS [2], by contrast, are quite similar but accept fasciculations alone as evidence of active denervation

ALS amyotrophic lateral sclerosis, *EMG* electromyography, *UMN* upper motor neurons, *LMN* lower motor neurons

cells, nerve roots, and peripheral nerve, as well as in some normal individuals, are often prominent as well. Nerve conduction studies and electromyography should always be performed in order to confirm lower motor neuron involvement, to determine the extent of lower motor neuron involvement, and to exclude other neuromuscular causes of weakness such as polyneuropathy, disorders of neuromuscular transmission, and myopathy. Often needle electromyography provides evidence of loss of lower motor neurons in muscles with normal bulk and strength. Conversely, in some cases the clinical presentation may be so striking that NCS/EMG hardly seems necessary; however, the consequences of making a diagnosis of ALS are so profound that a careful search for other causes of weakness is mandatory.

The Revised El Escorial criteria for the diagnosis of ALS incorporate the presence of upper motor neuron signs, lower motor neuron signs, and electrodiagnostic evidence of lower motor neuron disease into diagnostic categories of possible, probable, and definite ALS (Table 4.1) [1]. The El Escorial criteria divide the body into four regions (cranial, cervical, thoracic, and lumbosacral) and base the terms "possible, probable, and definite" ALS upon the number of regions (one, two, or three, respectively) affected. That said, in many cases the clinical findings are geographically restricted to one or two regions at the time of initial presentation but are nonetheless unequivocal. In such cases, when alternative etiologies of the findings are reasonably excluded, one can be confident of the diagnosis of ALS even though the El Escorial classification is only "possible" or "probable." The King's staging system is an ALS staging paradigm based upon the geographical extent of functional deficits and the presence of disease milestones [3].

ALS Mimics

There are a handful of conditions most likely to be misdiagnosed as ALS. These include the following:

• Structural lesions of the spinal cord or brainstem

Any lesion that damages lower motor neurons in the brainstem or anterior horn will result in lower motor neuron findings (Fig. 4.2). The clue, of course, is that the lower motor neuron findings will be present *only* at the level of the lesion. If the lesion also affects the corticospinal tracts at this level, upper motor neuron findings will be present below the level of the lesion. For this reason, whenever lower motor neuron findings exist exclusively rostral to upper motor neuron findings, imaging (usually MRI) of the relevant level of the central nervous system is mandatory. Cervical spondylosis, meningioma, and syrinx are among the many lesions that might result in such a presentation.

• Inclusion body myositis

Inclusion body myositis is a slowly progressive myopathy of older adults, which, because of the presence of atrophy, weakness without sensory findings, and largely preserved reflexes, is occasionally mistaken for ALS. The distinction is made on the basis of a distinctive distribution of muscle weakness, absence of pathologic reflexes, myopathic features on EMG, and characteristic findings on muscle biopsy. IBM is discussed in more detail in the chapter on myopathies.

• Spinobulbar muscular atrophy (SBMA or Kennedy's disease)

SBMA is an X-linked disease of lower motor neurons with prominent bulbar involvement. It is discussed further below.

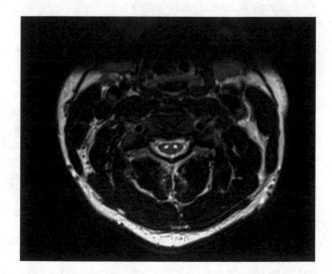

Fig. 4.2 Cervical MRI demonstrating high signal in anterior horn in patient presenting with lower motor neuron findings mimicking ALS

- Multifocal motor neuropathy

Multifocal motor neuropathy (MMN) is a pure motor condition often associated with prominent fasciculations, leading to occasional confusion with ALS. Unlike ALS, pathologic reflexes are not present in MMN; furthermore, MMN tends to present in the distribution of individual nerves rather than spinal cord segments and is diagnosed on the basis of distinctive electrodiagnostic features that are usually readily identified. MMN responds well to immunotherapy, so it is important not to miss the diagnosis. MMN is discussed in more detail in the chapter on neuropathies.

- Distal hereditary motor neuropathy (dHMN)

dHMN is a genetically determined motor neuropathy that presents with progressive distal-predominant weakness and atrophy over several years' time, much like other more common forms of CMT. Unlike other forms of CMT, there is no sensory involvement. Unlike ALS, in most forms of dHMN, there are no upper motor neuron signs. At times it can be difficult to distinguish dHMN in a patient with relatively brisk reflexes from ALS with predominantly lower motor neuron involvement, particularly as either can present with or without a compelling family history.

ALS Subtypes

ALS typically begins focally and spreads to adjacent regions (Fig. 4.3). Limb weakness is the initial symptom in about 70% of people with ALS (*limb-onset ALS*), while dysarthria or dysphagia (*bulbar-onset ALS*) is the initial symptom in about 25% of people with ALS. Rarely (about 5%) the initial symptom is truncal weakness or ventilatory dysfunction [4].

The following can be considered distinct forms of ALS:

- Progressive bulbar palsy (PBP)

PBP is a term often applied to a form of bulbar-onset ALS that progresses to severe bulbar dysfunction, with loss of useful speech and usually profound dysphagia, before any functionally significant limb weakness develops.

- Brachial amyotrophic diplegia (BAD)

BAD is an ALS subtype in which flaccid paralysis of both upper limbs progresses long before patients develop significant weakness of cranial, thoracic, or lumbosacral segments [5]. People with this subtype generally survive longer than people with other forms of ALS but require complete assistance in many activities of daily living because they cannot use their upper limbs. Leg amyotrophic diplegia (LAD) is a rare lower limb variant [6].

- Progressive muscular atrophy (PMA)

PMA refers to a pure or predominantly lower motor neuron syndrome, in which clear upper motor neuron signs may never develop, but which progresses inexorably in the same fashion as ALS and is not currently recognized as having a distinct etiology.

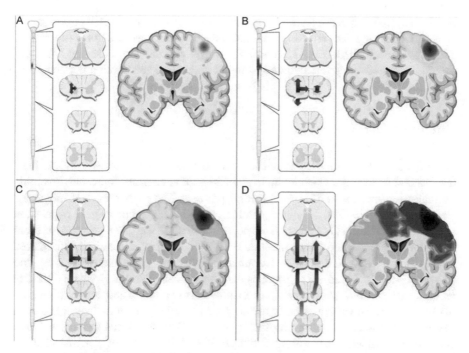

Fig. 4.3 Classic diagram from Ravits and La Spada illustrating the hypothesis that ALS begins in corresponding upper and lower motor neuron pools (A) and then generally progresses to motor neuron pools with anatomic proximity to those previously affected (B through D) in both cortical and bulbospinal regions. (Reproduced with permission from Wolters Kluwer Health) [7]

Unlike PLS, PMA does lead to ventilatory failure because lower motor neuron loss leads to weakness. Particular care must be taken in the diagnostic process to exclude motor neuropathy or myopathy in people presenting without upper motor neuron signs.

Cognitive and Behavioral Dysfunction and ALS

Forty to 50% of people with ALS demonstrate cognitive or behavioral impairment on validated assessments of these domains. In about 10% of cases, the deficits are sufficiently severe to fulfill criteria for frontotemporal dementia (FTD) [8, 9]. The deficits vary among individuals, presenting with a wide variety of problems such as impulsivity, loss of social empathy, disinhibition, or perseverative behaviors [10].

In addition to a full psychometric battery, validated instruments designed specifically to assess cognitive and behavioral deficits in ALS include the Edinburgh Cognitive Assessment Scale (ECAS) [11] and the ALS Cognitive Behavioral Screen (ALS CBS) [12].

Pseudobulbar affect (PBA) is common in ALS and is particularly prevalent among individuals with bulbar-onset ALS, progressive bulbar palsy, and FTD. PBA is a form of laughter or crying which is precipitated by appropriate social triggers but distinct in that it is excessive, uncontrollable, and stereotyped in its appearance; an experienced clinician can easily distinguish PBA from normal emotional expression. The prevalence of PBA in ALS and FTD may represent evidence that these are disorders of cortical systems related to social interaction and communication.

Etiology of ALS

A unifying etiology for ALS is not known. In recent years, however, it has been demonstrated that cytoplasmic inclusions in motor neurons represent insoluble ubiquitinated inclusions of one of several proteins. The most prevalent molecular structure is TDP-43 [13], a nuclear protein involved in regulation of gene expression and RNA stabilization, but others have been described as well. The presence of these inclusions has spawned some theories of ALS pathogenesis, including impaired RNA function, impaired protein degradation pathways, prion-like templating, and spread of pathologic protein aggregates from cell to cell. Neuronal hyperexcitability resulting in excitotoxicity, pathology in non-neuronal cells, and immune mechanisms, as well as a variety of other metabolic and oxidative disturbances, have been identified as possible contributing factors as well [14]. As of this writing, a single common mechanism for motor neuron death in ALS has not been demonstrated.

Numerous mutations, including mutations in the TDP-43 gene itself, have been identified as causes of familial ALS. The single most common genetic cause of familial ALS, responsible for 40–50% of people with ALS and a positive family history and 7–9% of people with ALS with a negative family history, is an expanded hexanucleotide repeat sequence in the C9orf72 gene [15]. This repeat expansion is also a recognized cause of FTD, and either ALS or FTD might be the presenting diagnosis of different individuals in the same family. The identification of a known cause of familial ALS in a substantial proportion of patients otherwise identified as having sporadic ALS (i.e., without a family history of the disease) [16] suggests a genetic role in a larger proportion of "sporadic" cases than had previously been recognized.

Management of ALS

ALS clinics have established the model for multidisciplinary care in neurodegenerative disease. The American Academy of Neurology has outlined management recommendations for the care of people living with ALS via a practice guideline and quality measure statement [17, 18]. Care of the person living with ALS spans numerous domains, including the following (Table 4.2) [4]. Many are described in greater detail in the chapters on rehabilitation management and ventilatory management.

- Ventilatory function: pulmonary function is monitored routinely and both noninvasive and invasive mechanical ventilation offered when indicated.

Table 4.2 Multidisciplinary management of ALS

Problem	Management	Expert team member
Ventilatory impairment	Noninvasive ventilation Tracheostomy with mechanical ventilation	Respiratory therapist Pulmonologist
Weak cough	Manually assisted cough Lung volume recruitment Mechanically assisted cough (insufflator/exsufflator)	Respiratory therapist
Dysarthria	Augmentative communication devices	Speech/language pathologist
Dysphagia	Dietary modifications Gastrostomy	Speech/language pathologist
Sialorrhea	Anticholinergic medications Botulinum toxin to salivary glands Radiation therapy to salivary glands	Neurologist
Weight loss	High-calorie, high-fat diet Estimating caloric needs based upon activity	Registered dietician
Impaired ADLs	Adaptations, equipment	Occupational therapist
Impaired mobility and falls	Gait aids, wheelchair, power chair	Physical therapist
Spasticity	Stretching, oral baclofen, tizanidine, dantrolene, and intrathecal baclofen	Neurologist or physical medicine and rehabilitation specialist
Pain	Physical therapy, medications	Neurologist, physical therapist, pain medicine specialist
Anxiety, depression, and changing life roles	Counseling, medications	Psychologist, neurologist
Pseudobulbar affect	Dextromethorphan/quinidine (Nuedexta®), amitriptyline	Neurologist
Cognitive and behavioral impairment, dementia	Screening instruments, diagnostic instruments, safety evaluations	Occupational therapist, neuropsychologist
Life planning	Financial counseling, advance directive, POLST	Social worker, attorney, neurologist
Clinical research	Discussion, online resources	Neurologist, research coordinator, patient advocacy group representative

In addition to the needs listed, patient advocacy groups such as ALS Association and Muscular Dystrophy Association (USA), Motor Neuron Disease Association (UK), and others provide numerous services including clinic certification and funding, care services and education directly to patients and families, research funding, advocacy, and support groups

POLST provider orders for life-sustaining treatment, *ALS* amyotrophic lateral sclerosis

- Cough effectiveness: peak cough flow and maximal expiratory pressure correlate with cough effectiveness; ineffective cough can be managed with manually assisted coughing, insufflator-exsufflator, and lung volume recruitment.
- Dysarthria: a broad range of augmentative communication devices is available when speech becomes ineffective.
- Dysphagia: swallowing needs to be reevaluated regularly and dietary recommendations made. Gastrostomy is indicated when nutritional needs cannot be met safely because of dysphagia. Because the procedure carries increased risk in people with malnutrition or hypoventilation, gastrostomy is often performed prior to need.
- Sialorrhea: dysphagia impairs physiologic clearance of saliva, resulting in drooling. There are several treatment options for this troublesome symptom.
- Weight loss: in addition to loss of muscle bulk, people with ALS lose weight from dysphagia, eating fatigue, loss of appetite, and increased energy expenditure due to clumsy or ineffective walking, transferring, and activities of daily living.
- Activities of daily living are affected dramatically by ALS and are discussed in detail in the chapter on rehabilitation management.
- Mobility and fall prevention are discussed in detail in the chapter on rehabilitation management.
- Spasticity: stretching, oral agents, and intrathecal baclofen are used to manage spasticity in ALS.
- Sleep: sleep efficiency is impacted by sleep-disordered breathing, difficulty turning, and anxiety. Poor sleep exacerbates fatigue in ALS.
- Medical complications of immobility include pain, adhesive capsulitis, deep vein thrombosis, atelectasis, skin breakdown, and constipation.
- Anxiety and depression.
- Life planning includes planning for retirement or disability, financial planning, and end-of-life planning.
- Engagement in research: clinic visits provide an opportunity for providers and research coordinators to educate people with ALS regarding opportunities to participate in clinical research.

Riluzole has demonstrated efficacy in slowing progression of disease [19]. Designed to alleviate glutamate-mediated excitotoxicity, riluzole has a modest but reproducibly demonstrated benefit. Edaravone has demonstrated slowing of progression of functional deficit in a subset of people with ALS [20].

End of Life Care

People with ALS die of ventilatory failure and make individual decisions regarding the degree of ventilatory support they desire based upon their assessment of their quality of life at the time such needs arise. Planning for end of life care and completion of an advanced directive (AD) and Provider Orders for Life-Sustaining Treatment (POLST) can ease the process of care for people with advanced ALS, but it is important for providers to readdress advanced directives periodically, as circumstances and decisions can change (Fig. 4.4) (Case 4.1).

MINNESOTA **Provider Orders for Life-Sustaining Treatment (POLST)**

Follow these orders until orders change. These medical orders are based on the patient's current medical conditions and preferences. Any action not completed does not invalidate the form and implies full treatment for that section. With significant change of condition new orders may need to be written. Patients should always be treated with dignity and respect.

LAST NAME | FIRST NAME | MEDICAL INITIAL

DATE OF BIRTH

PRIMARY MEDICAL CARE PROVIDER NAME   PRIMARY MEDICAL CARE PROVIDER PHONE (WITH AREA CODE)

A
CHECK ONE

CARDIOPULMONARY RESUSCITATION (CPR) Patient has no pulse and is not breathing.
☐ Attempt Resuscitation / CPR (Note: selecting this requires selecting "Full Treatment" in Section B).
☐ Do Not Attempt Resuscitation / DNR (Allow Natural Death).
When not in cardiopulmonary arrest, follow orders in B.

B
CHECK ONE
(NOTE: REQUIRE-MENTS)

MEDICAL TREATMENTS Patient has pulse and/or is breathing.
☐ **Full Treatment.** Use intubation, advanced airway interventions, and mechanical ventilation as indicated. Transfer to hospital and/or intensive care unit if indicated. A1 patients will receive comfort-focused treatments.
TREATMENT PLAN: Full treatment including life support measures in the intensive care unit.
☐ **Selective Treatment.** Use medical treatment, antibiotics, IV fluids and cardiac monitor as indicated. No intubation, advanced airway interventions, or mechanical ventilation. May consider less invasive airway support (e.g. CPAP, BiPAP). Transfer to hospital if indicated. Generally avoid the intensive care unit. All patients will receive comfort-focused treatments.
TREATMENT PLAN: Provide basic medical treatments aimed at treating new or reversible illness.
☐ **Comfort-Focused Treatment (Allow Natural Death).** Relieve pain and suffering through the use of any medication by any route, positioning, wound care and other measures. Use oxygen, suction and manual treatment of airway obstruction as needed for comfort. Patient prefers no transfer to hospital for life-sustaining treatments. Transfer if comfort needs cannot be met in current location.
TREATMENT PLAN: Maximize comfort through symptom management.

C
CHECK ALL THAT APPLY

DOCUMENTATION OF DISCUSSION
☐ Patient (Patient has capacity)   ☐ Other Surrogate
☐ Court-Appointed Guardian   ☐ Health Care Agent
☐ Parent of Minor   ☐ Health Care Directive

NAME (PRINT)

PHONE (WITH AREA CODE)

SIGNATURE OF PATIENT OR SURROGATE

D

SIGNATURE OF PHYSICIAN / APRN / PA
My signature below indicates to the best of my knowledge that these orders are consistent with the patient's current medical conditions and preferences.

SIGNATURE (STRONGLY RECOMMENDED)

RELATIONSHIP (IF YOU ARE THE PATIENT, WRITE "SELF")

Signature attests to above that these orders reflect the patient's treatment wishes. Absence of signature does not negate the above orders.

NAME (PRINT) (REQUIRED)   LICENSE TYPE (REQUIRED)   PHONE (WITH AREA CODE)

SIGNATURE (REQUIRED)   DATE (REQUIRED)

SEND FORM WITH PATIENT WHENEVER TRANSFERRED OR DISCHARGED. FAXED, PHOTOCOPIED OR ELECTRONIC VERSIONS OF THIS FORM ARE VALID.

Minnesota Provider Orders for Life-Sustaining Treatment (POLST)   www.polstmn.org   PAGE 1 OF 2
521221- Rev 5/22/17   Advance Directives and Living Will   ORIGINAL: Patient   PHOTOCOPY: To Medical Record

---

INFORMATION FOR

PATIENT NAMED ON THIS FORM

E
CHECK ONE FROM EACH SECTION

ADDITIONAL PATIENT PREFERENCES (OPTIONAL)

ARTIFICIALLY ADMINISTERED NUTRITION Offer food by mouth if feasible.
☐ Long-term artificial nutrition by tube.
☐ Defined trial period of artificial nutrition by tube.
☐ No artificial nutrition by tube.

ANTIBIOTICS
☐ Use IV/IM antibiotic treatment.
☐ Oral antibiotics only (no IV/IM).
☐ No antibiotics. Use other methods to relieve symptoms when possible.

ADDITIONAL PATIENT PREFERENCES (e.g. dialysis, duration of intubation).

CLINICIAN WHO PREPARED DOCUMENT ☐ check if same as MD/APRN/PA signing on front

PREPARER NAME (REQUIRED)   PREPARER TITLE (REQUIRED)

PREPARER PHONE (WITH AREA CODE) (REQUIRED)   DATE PREPARED (REQUIRED)

NOTE TO PATIENTS AND SURROGATES
The POLST form is always voluntary and is for persons with advanced illness or frailty. POLST records your wishes for medical treatment in your current state of health. Once initial medical treatment is begun and the risks and benefits of further therapy are clear, your treatment wishes may change. Your medical care and this form can be changed to reflect your new wishes at any time. However, no form can address all the medical treatment decisions that may need to be made.

DIRECTIONS FOR HEALTH CARE PROVIDERS
Completing POLST
• Completing a POLST is always voluntary and cannot be mandated for a patient.
• POLST should reflect current preferences of persons with advanced illness or frailty. Also, encourage completion of a Health Care Directive.
• Verbal / phone orders are acceptable with follow-up signature by physician/APRN/PA in accordance with facility/community policy.
• A surrogate may include a court-appointed guardian, Health Care Agent designated in a Health Care Directive, or a person whom the patient's health care provider believes best knows what is in the patient's best interest and will make decision in accordance with the patient's expressed wishes and values to the extent known, such as a verbally designated surrogate, spouse, registered domestic partner, parent of a minor, or closest available relative.

Reviewing POLST
This POLST should be reviewed periodically, and if:
• The patient is transferred from one care setting or care level to another, or
• There is a substantial change in the patient's health status, or
• The patient's treatment preferences change, or
• The patient's Primary Medical Care Provider changes.

Voiding POLST
• A person with capacity, or the valid surrogate of a person without capacity, can void the form and request alternative treatment.
• Draw line through sections A through E and write "VOID" in large letters if POLST is replaced or becomes invalid.
• If included in an electronic medical record, follow voiding procedures of facility/community.

A Health Care Directive is recommended for all capable adults, regardless of their health status. A Health Care Directive allows you to document in detail your future health care instructions and/or name a Health Care Agent to speak for you if you are unable to speak for yourself.

SEND FORM WITH PATIENT WHENEVER TRANSFERRED OR DISCHARGED. FAXED, PHOTOCOPIED OR ELECTRONIC VERSIONS OF THIS FORM ARE VALID.

Minnesota Provider Orders for Life-Sustaining Treatment (POLST)   www.polstmn.org   PAGE 2 OF 2
521221- Rev 5/22/17   Advance Directives and Living Will   ORIGINAL: Patient   PHOTOCOPY: To Medical Record

Fig. 4.4 For those who choose to limit aggressive intervention in the case of an acute medical deterioration, the POLST (Provider Orders for Life-Sustaining Treatment) summarizes their wishes in the form of a provider's order to emergency personnel. While first responders still have some latitude in addressing emergencies as circumstances dictate, the POLST translates a person's wishes, which are usually documented more fully in an advanced directive, into clear and succinct medical orders

Case 4.1

A 64-year-old man presented with a 9-month history of weakness at the right ankle. Two months after onset he had undergone a lumbar discectomy for presumed compressive radiculopathy. Despite surgery his weakness did not improve, and his wife felt it may have worsened since surgery. He had fallen once after tripping on a rug. He denied back pain or sensory loss. Review of systems was also positive for muscle cramps in bilateral lower and right upper limbs. Family history was unremarkable.

Neurologic examination revealed normal mental status, cranial nerve, and sensory examinations. Motor examination demonstrated 4+/5 strength of right finger extensors, interossei, and thumb abduction. In the lower limbs, ankle dorsiflexion was 4/5 on the right and 4+/5 on the left, with mild atrophy noted only in the right first dorsal interosseous and right tibialis anterior muscles. Tone was normal. Reflexes were absent at the jaw, brisk in bilateral upper limbs with spread to finger flexors from biceps and brachioradialis, and brisk in the lower limbs with a probable extensor plantar response on the right only. A Hoffmann's sign was present on the right as well.

Spinal imaging demonstrated a disk bulge at C6–C7 with mild and moderate narrowing of the neural foramina on the right and left, respectively, and adequate postoperative resolution of right L5 root compression. Nerve conduction studies demonstrated normal sensory conduction studies and a reduced right peroneal compound muscle action potential amplitude and were otherwise normal. Electromyography demonstrated fibrillation potentials, fasciculation potentials, and long-duration, high-amplitude motor unit potentials with reduced recruitment in bilateral lower limbs and the right C7–T1 segments. Frequent fibrillation potentials were seen in thoracic paraspinal muscles as well. Pulmonary function studies were normal.

The patient was given a diagnosis of ALS. The diagnostic process, natural history, and management of ALS were discussed with him and his adult son. Options for management of ventilatory failure and the value of an advanced directive were discussed briefly. He chose to begin treatment with riluzole and edaravone. He met with a physical therapist to address falls prevention and the potential need for gait aids. He was informed of currently enrolling clinical research studies in ALS and registered with the ALS Association and Muscular Dystrophy Association.

The patient was next seen 6 months after his initial visit. In the interim he had experienced several falls and was developing difficulty writing with his dominant right hand. He was instructed in the use of a four-wheeled walker, which he declined to use. At that visit he underwent a screening assessment for cognitive impairment and scored in the range predicting mild cognitive impairment. His wife completed a screening instrument for behavioral impairment based upon her observations, and the result was in the normal range. He had not completed his advanced directive and indicated that was due in part to the fact that he was considering long-term mechanical ventilation but had not yet decided.

One year after his initial visit, he was ambulating principally with a walker. He was experiencing increased difficulty using his hands for self-care, writing, using utensils, and keyboarding. He noted mild slurring of speech when tired but no difficulty swallowing. Pulmonary function remained normal.

One and a half years after his initial visit, he was no longer ambulatory. He was increasingly dependent upon family for help with activities of daily living, due to both upper and lower extremity weakness. Family were taking turns caring for him as his wife was recovering from breast cancer treatment and was too frail to provide more than minimal assistance to him. Their oldest daughter had taken a leave from work and moved from another state to help in his care. On examination, in addition to limb weakness, he had a mixed dysarthria, but speech was fully comprehensible. A cognitive and behavioral screening instrument again predicted cognitive impairment but not dementia. His family reported no observed cognitive or behavioral change from baseline other than modest irritability. The patient refused psychometric assessment. He had moderate dysphagia for thin liquids and was placed on a dysphagia diet. He had lost 20 pounds. Pulmonary function studies were clearly abnormal for the first time, with a forced vital capacity of 64%, maximal inspiratory pressure of −50, and maximal expiratory pressure of 30. Cough was weak. Gastrostomy was recommended based upon the combined evidence of developing dysphagia and progressive loss of ventilatory function. He was referred for an augmentative communication evaluation and initiation of nocturnal noninvasive ventilation (NIV) and was provided an insufflator-exsufflator (cough assist device). The patient's goals of care were discussed. He indicated that he did not want to undergo gastrostomy and had decided against long-term mechanical ventilation but did want to receive treatment for reversible medical conditions. A POLST was completed at that time.

Two years after his initial visit, the patient was unable to use his upper limbs to assist in ADLs. He was hospitalized with increasing dyspnea, secretions, and fever despite the use of noninvasive ventilation and cough assist. Chest X-ray demonstrated a right lower lobe infiltrate and he was treated for pneumonia. Symptoms improved, and he was discharged to home, where he enrolled in hospice shortly thereafter.

Two and a half years after his initial visit, the patient passed away at home.

Discussion: This is a representative example of just a few of the management issues in ALS. Disability often progresses faster than a person with ALS is prepared to adjust; hence, numerous decisions, from adoption of gait aids, timing of gastrostomy, or life planning decisions, are sometimes made only after the problem becomes critically time-sensitive. Physical, emotional, and financial burdens on caregivers are considerable. Cognitive impairment, behavioral impairment, and mood disorders, even when they are not sufficiently severe to remove decision-making capacity and autonomy, compound these problems.

Progression of disease can be measured in many ways. The ALS Functional Rating Scale-Revised (ALSFRS-R) is a well-established and validated method to chart progression in bulbar, upper limb (fine motor, ADLs), trunk and lower limb (gross motor, mobility), and ventilatory domains [21]. Figure 4.5 is an example of disease progression along all these parameters.

Milestones, such as loss of useful speech, loss of independent ambulation, placement of gastrostomy or initiation of noninvasive ventilation, and death or need for continuous ventilatory assistance, represent important clinical outcomes as well. The aforementioned can be mapped to clinical stages using the King's or other staging criteria. Finally, ventilatory parameters and weight represent clinical data with important prognostic significance.

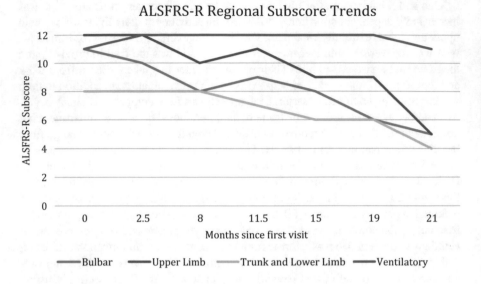

Fig. 4.5 Example of progression of ALSFRS-R total score and subscores over time. This is a common outcome measure in ALS clinical trials and can be used clinically to measure rate of change and to map to the King's ALS stage. ALSFRS-R also gives the clinician a "snapshot" of the domains and severity of a person's functional disability and, by extension, their speech, occupational, physical, and respiratory therapy needs

Primary Lateral Sclerosis

Primary lateral sclerosis (PLS) is a progressive degenerative disorder of upper motor neurons alone. While there is some controversy as to whether PLS is distinct from ALS or represents ALS with only minimal, subclinical lower motor neuron involvement, it is distinct in that there is no substantial effect on life expectancy because ventilatory failure in ALS reflects weakness due to loss of lower motor neurons innervating the diaphragm and accessory muscles of ventilation. While ALS can present with little or no lower motor neuron involvement at onset, PLS diagnostic criteria require the absence of lower motor neuron signs 3 or 4 years after onset [22, 23]. The cause of PLS is not known, and management consists largely of management of spasticity and its functional consequences.

Spinal Muscular Atrophy

Spinal muscular atrophy (SMA) is an autosomal recessive disorder presenting with progressive, symmetric, proximal-predominant weakness in infancy, childhood, or adulthood. It is a pure lower motor neuron syndrome and is due to homozygous deletion or mutation of the SMN1 gene, which is named as an acronym for survival of the motor neuron because of the consequences of its deletion. The severity of the phenotype reflects the number of available copies of the SMN2 gene, which produces a similar but less stable protein. Management of SMA has been revolutionized by approval of an antisense oligonucleotide designed to produce a stable copy of the SMN protein [24]. SMA is discussed in detail in Chap. 6.

Spinobulbar Muscular Atrophy or Kennedy's Disease

Spinobulbar muscular atrophy (SBMA) is a multisystem disorder caused by a repeat expansion in the androgen receptor gene on the X chromosome [25]. It causes mild androgen insensitivity, resulting in mild to moderate gynecomastia and reduced fertility in males. The more clinically evident problems due to this diagnosis are a lower motor neuron disease with universal involvement of the bulbar musculature as well as the limbs. A mild distal sensory neuropathy is present as well. Patients typically present with a flaccid dysarthria, dysphagia, and slowly progressive limb weakness. Physical findings, in addition to gynecomastia, include tongue and facial fasciculations; tongue atrophy; atrophy of extremity muscles, usually with prominent upper limb involvement; tremor; and mild sensory loss in the distal lower limbs [26]. Upper motor neuron signs are absent. Symptoms and signs can emerge during puberty, but many patients do not present until mid-adult life. Ventilatory function is often compromised, but death due to ventilatory failure is rare. The precise mechanism of motor neuron and sensory axon injury is unknown, and as yet care is supportive.

Poliomyelitis

Poliomyelitis is an acute and irreversible disease of lower motor neurons due to viral, usually enteroviral, infections. The syndrome of acute poliomyelitis therefore begins with a viral gastroenteritis, followed by rapidly progressive segmental cramps, fasciculations, and weakness. Lumbar puncture reveals a pleocytosis and elevated CSF protein consistent with an acute infectious illness. While the virus that is named for the disease is largely eradicated, acute poliomyelitis rarely occurs after infection with other enteroviruses or after West Nile virus infection.

Hirayama Disease (Monomelic Amyotrophy)

Monomelic amyotrophy, or Hirayama disease, is a rare focal motor neuron disease with a stereotyped clinical course. It typically presents with very gradually progressive weakness and atrophy in the hand which is unilateral or, less commonly,

a   b

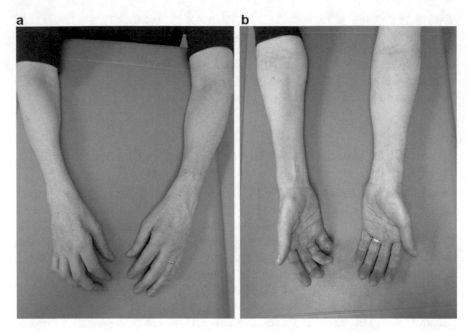

Fig. 4.6 Asymmetric upper limb atrophy as seen in monomelic atrophy. Note atrophy of forearm muscles and first dorsal interosseous muscle on the patient's right upper limb

bilateral but asymmetric (Fig. 4.6). Over a period of years, it progresses in severity until the hand is severely weak (antigravity or weaker) and atrophic and progresses in extent to involve distal forearm muscles. It does not extend beyond this region. Upper motor neuron signs are not present. Monomelic amyotrophy presents almost exclusively in males in their late teens or twenties. It is distinguished from lower trunk plexopathy by the absence of clinical or electrophysiologic evidence of sensory involvement and is distinguished from ALS by the slow progression, restricted geographic extent, and absence of upper motor neuron signs. MR imaging of the cervical spine demonstrates high T2 signal, indicative of gliosis, in the anterior horn and often demonstrates atrophy of the lower cervical cord as well. While this can be seen with other causes of anterior cervical myelopathy such as spondylotic myelopathy, the specific imaging correlate of Hirayama disease is seen with cervical imaging during neck flexion (dynamic MRI; Fig. 4.7). In Hirayama disease dynamic MRI demonstrates anterior displacement of the posterior dura and compression of the spinal cord between the vertebral bodies anteriorly and the dura posteriorly. The potential space posterior to the cord is filled by epidural fat and engorged dural venous plexus, but the presumed mechanism of Hirayama disease is insufficient laxity of the posterior dura, such that it becomes taut and compresses the spinal cord in flexion [27]. The postulated mechanism of injury is compression of the anterior spinal artery and selective vascular vulnerability of the anterior horns.

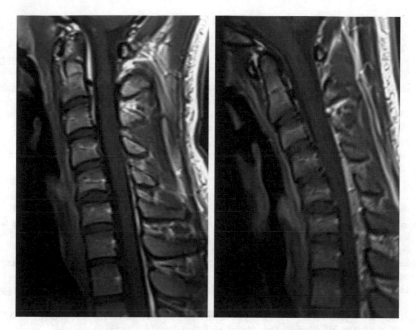

Fig. 4.7 Dynamic MRI demonstrating compression of cervical cord in flexion in Hirayama disease

Summary

Motor neuron disorders should be considered in any patient presenting with a pure motor disorder and atrophy. The most common acquired motor neuron disorder is ALS, which usually presents with symptoms restricted to the limb, bulbar, truncal, or ventilatory muscles and subsequently spreads to other regions. Clinicians should also be familiar with PLS, SBMA, monomelic amyotrophy, and poliomyelitis. Important mimics of ALS and other motor neuron diseases include structural lesions affecting lower motor neurons in the brainstem and spinal cord, IBM, and MMN.

References

1. Brooks BR, Miller RG, Swash M, Munsat TL. World Federation of Neurology Research Group on Motor Neuron D. El Escorial revisited: revised criteria for the diagnosis of amyotrophic lateral sclerosis. Amyotroph Lateral Scler Other Motor Neuron Disord. 2000;1(5):293–9.
2. de Carvalho M, Dengler R, Eisen A, England JD, Kaji R, Kimura J, et al. Electrodiagnostic criteria for diagnosis of ALS. Clin Neurophysiol. 2008;119(3):497–503.
3. Balendra R, Jones A, Jivraj N, Knights C, Ellis CM, Burman R, et al. Estimating clinical stage of amyotrophic lateral sclerosis from the ALS Functional Rating Scale. Amyotroph Lateral Scler Frontotemporal Degener. 2014;15(3–4):279–84.
4. Kiernan MC, Vucic S, Cheah BC, Turner MR, Eisen A, Hardiman O, et al. Amyotrophic lateral sclerosis. Lancet. 2011;377(9769):942–55.

5. Katz JS, Wolfe GI, Andersson PB, Saperstein DS, Elliott JL, et al. Brachial amyotrophic diplegia: a slowly progressive motor neuron disorder. Neurology. 1999;53:1071–6.
6. Dimachkie MM, Muzyka IM, Katz JS, Jackson C, Wang Y, et al. Leg amyotrophic diplegia: prevalence and pattern of weakness at US neuromuscular centers. J Clin Neuromuscul Dis. 2013;15:7–12.
7. Ravits J, La Spada A. ALS motor phenotype heterogeneity, focality and spread: deconstructing motor neuron degeneration. Neurology 2009;73:805–811.
8. Giordana MT, Ferrero P, Grifoni S, Pellerino A, Naldi A, Montuschi A. Dementia and cogni- tive impairment in amyotrophic lateral sclerosis: a review. Neurol Sci. 2011;32(1):9–16.
9. Murphy J, Factor-Litvak P, Goetz R, Lomen-Hoerth C, Nagy PL, Hupf J, et al. Cognitive-behavioral screening reveals prevalent impairment in a large multicenter ALS cohort. Neurology. 2016;86(9):813–20.
10. Waldo ML. The frontotemporal dementias. Psychiatr Clin North Am. 2015;38(2):193–209.
11. Abrahams S, Newton J, Niven E, Foley J, Bak TH. Screening for cognition and behaviour changes in ALS. Amyotroph Lateral Scler Frontotemporal Degener. 2014;15(1–2):9–14.
12. Woolley SC, York MK, Moore DH, Strutt AM, Murphy J, Schulz PE, et al. Detecting frontotemporal dysfunction in ALS: utility of the ALS Cognitive Behavioral Screen (ALS-CBS). Amyotroph Lateral Scler. 2010;11(3):303–11.
13. Saberi S, Stauffer JE, Schulte DJ, Ravits J. Neuropathology of amyotrophic lateral sclerosis and its variants. Neurol Clin. 2015;33:855–76.
14. Peters OM, Ghasemi M, Brown RH Jr. Emerging mechanisms of molecular pathology in ALS. J Clin Invest. 2015;125(5):1767–79.
15. Ji A-L, Zhang X, Chen W-W, Huang W-J. Genetic insight into the amyotrophic lateral sclerosis/frontotemporal dementia spectrum. J Med Genet. 2017;54:145–54.
16. Majounie E, Renton AE, Mok K, Dopper EG, Waite A, Rollinson S, et al. Frequency of the C9orf72 hexanucleotide repeat expansion in patients with amyotrophic lateral sclerosis and frontotemporal dementia: a cross-sectional study. Lancet Neurol. 2012;11(4):323–30.
17. Miller RG, Jackson CE, Kasarskis EJ, England JD, Forshew D, Johnston W, et al. Practice parameter update: the care of the patient with amyotrophic lateral sclerosis: multidisciplinary care, symptom management, and cognitive/behavioral impairment (an evidence-based review): report of the quality standards Subcommittee of the American Academy of Neurology. Neurology. 2009;73(15):1227–33.
18. Miller RG, Brooks BR, Swain-Eng RJ, Basner RC, Carter GT, Casey P, et al. Quality improvement in neurology: amyotrophic lateral sclerosis quality measures. Report of the quality measurement and reporting Subcommittee of the American Academy of Neurology. Amyotroph Lateral Scler Frontotemporal Degener. 2014;15(3–4):165–8.
19. Besimon G, Lacomplez L, Meininger V. A controlled trial of riluzole in amyotrophic lateral sclerosis and the ALS/Riluzole Study Group. N Engl J Med. 1994;330:585–91.
20. Edaravone (MC-186) ALS 19 study writing group. Safety and efficacy of edaravone in well defined patients with amyotrophic lateral sclerosis: a randomised, double-blind, placebo-controlled trial. Lancet Neurol 2017(16):505–512.
21. Cedarbaum JM, Stambler N, Malta E, Fuller C, Hilt D, et al. The ALSFRS-R: a revised functional rating scale that incorporates assessments of respiratory function. J Neurol Sci. 1999;169:13–21.
22. Pringle CE, Hudson AJ, Munoz DG, Kiernan JA, Brown WF, Ebers GC. Primary lateral sclerosis. Clinical features, neuropathology and diagnostic criteria. Brain. 1992;115(Pt 2):495–520.
23. Singer MA, Statland JM, Wolfe GI, Barohn RJ. Primary lateral sclerosis. Muscle Nerve. 2007;35(3):291–302.
24. Finkel RS, Mercuri E, Darras BT, Connolly AM, Kuntz NL, et al. Nusinersen versus sham control in infantile-onse spinal muscular atrophy. N Engl J Med. 2017;377:1723–32.
25. La Spada, A. Spinal and bulbar muscular atrophy. In: Pagon RA, Adam M, Ardinger HH, et al, editors. GeneReviews. Seattle: University of Washington; 2017.
26. Kennedy WR, Alter M, Sung JH. Progressive proximal spinal and bulbar muscular atrophy of late onset: a sex-linked recessive trait. Neurology 1968;18:671–680.
27. Huang Y-L, Chen C-C. Hirayama disease. Neuroimag Clin N Am. 2011;21:939–50.

Chapter 5
Diseases of Nerve

Jeffrey A. Allen

Abbreviations

AIDP	Acute inflammatory demyelinating polyneuropathy
AMAN	Acute motor axonal neuropathy
AMSAN	Acute motor-sensory axonal neuropathy
ANS	Autonomic nervous system
CIDP	Chronic inflammatory demyelinating polyneuropathy
CMT	Charcot-Marie-Tooth
CMV	Cytomegalovirus
CSF	Cerebrospinal fluid
CTS	Carpal tunnel syndrome
DADS	Distal acquired demyelinating symmetric neuropathy
DRG	Dorsal root ganglia
EMG	Electromyography
GBS	Guillain-Barré syndrome
HCV	Hepatitis C virus
HIV	Human immunodeficiency virus
HNPP	Hereditary liability to pressure palsies
MADSAM	Multifocal acquired sensory and motor neuropathy
MAG	Myelin-associated glycoprotein
MFS	Miller Fisher syndrome
MGUS	Monoclonal gammopathy of undetermined significance
MMN	Multifocal motor neuropathy
MRI	Magnetic resonance imaging
NCS	Nerve conduction studies
PLEX	Plasmapheresis
POEMS	Polyneuropathy, organomegaly, endocrinopathy, monoclonal gammopathy, and skin changes syndrome
TTR	Transthyretin
VEGF	Vascular endothelial growth factor

J.A. Allen, MD (✉)
Department of Neurology, University of Minnesota, Minneapolis, MN, USA
e-mail: jaallen@UMN.edu

© Springer International Publishing AG, part of Springer Nature 2018
D. Walk (ed.), *Clinical Handbook of Neuromuscular Medicine*,
https://doi.org/10.1007/978-3-319-67116-1_5

Key Points

- Positive sensory symptoms include paresthesias and allodynia, and positive motor symptoms may be cramps or fasciculations.
- Numbness is a negative sensory symptom, and weakness and atrophy are negative motor symptoms.
- The neurologic examination aims to define the type of modality affected, thereby establishing which type of nerve is affected.
- In length-dependent polyneuropathies, the ankle reflex is typically reduced, but more proximal reflexes are preserved. In generalized neuropathies reflexes are decreased in both proximal and distal areas.
- Polyneuropathies that affect only small fibers have normal reflexes.
- In length-dependent polyneuropathies, symptoms and signs are first recognized in the distal lower limbs.
- Evolving multiple mononeuropathies, especially when painful, should alert the clinician to the possibility of peripheral nerve vasculitis or peripheral nerve infiltrative disease.
- Acute and subacutely evolving neuropathies raise concern for an underlying inflammatory, dysimmune, or toxic cause.
- Symptoms from plexopathy typically include pain, weakness, and sensory loss in the distribution of the affected nerves within the plexus.
- Parsonage-Turner syndrome and diabetic amyotrophy both typically present with unilateral acute onset of pain followed by weakness and atrophy. In Parsonage-Turner syndrome, the upper limb is affected. In diabetic amyotrophy, the lower limb is affected and blood sugars are often (but not always) poorly controlled.
- When plexopathy is caused by a compressive or infiltrating mass (e.g., neoplasm, hematoma, abscess), pain often occurs early, with weakness and sensory deficits evolving later. Conversely, radiation-induced plexopathy most often leads to slowly worsening weakness and sensory change with a lesser pain component.
- Unilateral upper limb weakness after sternal retraction that clinically localizes to the medial cord and lower trunk is most likely due to stretching or avulsion of the lower portions of the brachial plexus, rather than acute stroke.
- Median nerve compression is the most commonly encountered compression neuropathy.
- Acute or subacute unilateral lower limb weakness that affects knee extension but spares foot dorsiflexion and thigh adduction raises concern for a femoral nerve injury. Especially if the patient is anticoagulated, retroperitoneal hematoma should be explored with imaging.
- Both peroneal neuropathy and L5 radiculopathy may result in ankle dorsiflexion and ankle eversion weakness. In peroneal neuropathy ankle inversion is normal, while in L5 radiculopathy ankle inversion may also be weak.
- Acute onset of pain, weakness, and sensory loss in a named nerve distribution are features that raise concern for peripheral nerve vasculitis.
- Lewis-Sumner syndrome and multifocal motor neuropathy are demyelinating neuropathies that are distinguished clinically from vasculitis by the typical

absence of pain at onset and from CIDP by the distribution of symptoms restricted to single or multiple named nerves.

- HNPP due to a PMP-22 deletion is a hereditary neuropathy that can mimic other acquired causes of mononeuropathy multiplex.
- Treatment for length-dependent axonal neuropathies is guided by the underlying condition.
- Progressive, symmetric, generalized (i.e., not length-dependent) polyneuropathies often show demyelination on nerve conduction studies and are pathophysiologically mediated by immune dysfunction.
- Early and frequent monitoring of pulmonary function is critical in GBS, as between 20 and 30% of patients develop respiratory failure and need mechanical ventilation in an intensive care unit.
- GBS treatment with either plasma exchange or IVIg should be initiated as soon as possible after diagnosis to prevent further nerve injury.
- Axonal GBS variants AMAN and especially AMSAN typically have a poorer prognosis than AIDP.
- The Miller Fisher syndrome variant of GBS typically has a better prognosis than AIDP, with most patients returning to full function within 3–5 months.
- CIDP is distinguished from GBS on clinical grounds by continued progression beyond 2 months.
- The DADS CIDP phenotype is associated with an IgM gammopathy in 2/3 of cases, and half of those also express anti-myelin-associated glycoprotein (MAG) antibodies.
- Although MMN classically shows conduction block on nerve conduction studies and about 50% have anti-GM1 ganglioside IgM antibodies, neither detectable conduction block nor GM1 antibodies are present in all patients with MMN.
- CMT1A due to PMP22 duplication is the most common hereditary peripheral neuropathy.
- CMT type 1 is demyelinating in pathophysiology, while CMT2 is axonal.
- POEMS refers to polyneuropathy, organomegaly, endocrinopathy, M protein, skin changes

Introduction

The peripheral nervous system (PNS) includes peripheral motor and sensory neurons, spinal nerves with their roots and rami, all cranial nerves except the optic nerve, and the peripheral components of the autonomic nervous system. When a pathologic process affects these components, either in a focal or generalized manner, the term peripheral neuropathy is often applied. In this chapter, unless otherwise indicated, the terms "peripheral neuropathy," "polyneuropathy," and "neuropathy" will be used interchangeably. Neuropathy should be suspected in any patient presenting with sensory and motor symptoms affecting more than one limb without signs referable to the central nervous system.

The potential causes of peripheral neuropathy are numerous. Although there is no single algorithm that best directs diagnostic testing, a fundamental understanding of the clinical deficits typical of peripheral neuropathy, the pattern of involvement, and potential causes can help the clinician craft an evaluation that is timely, accurate, and cost-effective [1, 2].

Symptoms and Signs of Peripheral Neuropathy

Certain clinical features support a diagnosis of peripheral neuropathy (Table 5.1).

Sensory and motor symptoms may be classified as either positive or negative. *Positive sensory symptoms* can be *spontaneous* and either painless (such as tingling) or painful (such as burning). They can be *stimulus-evoked*, such as with pain with light touch or pressure that is normally not painful (allodynia), or excessive pain with normally mildly painful stimuli (hyperalgesia). *Negative sensory symptoms* are an absence or reduction of sensory function (reduced tactile, thermal, or pain perception). *Positive motor symptoms* include fasciculations (muscle twitching) and cramps, while *negative motor symptoms and signs* include atrophy (loss of muscle bulk) and loss of power (weakness).

Small myelinated and unmyelinated fibers carry signals transduced from painful and thermal stimuli. Dysfunction of these "small fibers" often results in both positive and negative sensory symptoms and signs referable to these modalities. *Small fiber neuropathy* typically presents with prominent positive sensory symptoms such as spontaneous burning, paresthesias, sharp, shooting pains, and reduced or abnormal perception of pin and temperature. Large fiber dysfunction leads to faulty transmission of information from receptors involved in joint and limb position, vibration, and pressure. *Large fiber neuropathy* typically presents without prominent positive sensory symptoms but with loss of perception of touch, vibration, or joint position, and with loss of reflexes. *Imbalance, particularly in the dark or with eyes closed, is often a prominent symptom in large fiber neuropathy.*

Table 5.1 Symptoms and signs of peripheral neuropathy

Positive sensory symptoms, e.g., burning, tingling, "pins and needles"
Negative sensory symptoms, e.g., numbness
Positive motor symptoms, e.g., cramps and fasciculations
Negative motor symptoms, e.g., weakness and atrophy
Reduced or absent deep tendon reflexes
The distribution of symptoms and signs within a recognized peripheral nerve pattern, e.g., length-dependent, single nerve territory, multiple individual nerves, generalized
The absence of examination features implicating CNS involvement

Autonomic symptoms include orthostatic intolerance, syncope, diarrhea, consti-pation, early satiety, urinary complaints, erectile dysfunction, and abnormal sweat-ing. As some polyneuropathies that affect somatic nerves may also affect autonomic nerves, these symptoms are important to review with all patients. In practice, however, autonomic dysfunction due to polyneuropathy is uncommon. Autonomic neuropathy commonly occurs in neuropathy due to diabetes mellitus, particularly type 1, and neuropathy due to amyloidosis.

Reflexes are characteristically reduced (hyporeflexia) or absent (areflexia) in large fiber polyneuropathies. The distribution of reflex abnormalities is concordant with other aspects of the polyneuropathy pattern:

- In length-dependent polyneuropathies, the Achilles reflex is typically reduced, but more proximal reflexes are often preserved.
- In non-length-dependent neuropathies such as GBS or CIDP, reflexes are decreased at both proximal and distal sites.
- Reflexes are normal in patients with polyneuropathies that affect only small fibers.

Neuropathy Classification

To simplify the evaluation of neuropathy, neurologists classify neuropathies according to the following four features:

- *Distribution (length-dependent, non-length-dependent, or multifocal)*
- *Nature of the primary pathology (axonal or demyelinating)*
- *Modalities affected (motor, sensory large fiber, sensory small fiber, and autonomic)*
- *Time course*

Once characterized in this fashion, the differential diagnosis of a neuropathy is generally reduced to a manageable list of possibilities.

How does one determine these in clinical practice?

- The *distribution and modalities affected* can be determined largely from his-tory and examination and can be buttressed by EMG/NCS.
- To reliably determine the *nature of the primary pathology*, one needs electrodi-agnostic studies and rarely nerve biopsy as well, although experienced clinicians can often make an educated judgment regarding the pathologic process on the basis of clinical findings.
- The *time course* is generally self-evident.

Most neuropathies are chronic, involve both sensory and motor fibers to some degree, and conform to one of the patterns identified in Table 5.2.

Table 5.2 Distribution, pathology, and modalities affected for common categories of neuropathy. Detailed descriptions and key to abbreviations are provided in the text. Colors represent modalities affected, as follows: red, usually small fiber sensory-predominant; orange, small or large fiber sensory-predominant; green, sensorimotor; blue, motor-predominant; and violet, pure motor

	Length-dependent	Generalized (non-length-dependent)	Multifocal
Primary axonopathy	Metabolic Toxic Nutritional Infectious (HIV, HCV) CMT2 Idiopathic	Infiltrative AMAN AMSAN	Vasculitis Infiltrative
Primary myelinopathy	CMT1	CIDP (chronic) AIDP (acute)	MMN LSS

Temporal Evolution of Peripheral Neuropathy

The duration of symptoms can be somewhat arbitrarily defined as hyperacute (onset less than a few days), acute (days to 4 weeks), subacute (4–8 weeks), or chronic (more than 8 weeks). Generally speaking, *hyperacute* symptoms suggest traumatic or vasculitic pathophysiology, including that which can be seen in diabetic lumbo-sacral radiculoplexopathy and neuralgic amyotrophy (Parsonage-Turner syndrome). *Acute and subacutely evolving processes* include Guillain-Barré syndrome and its variants, toxic neuropathies, and vasculitic neuropathies, which as noted may initially appear hyperacute. Most length-dependent neuropathies are *chronic* and evolve slowly over years. Chronic inflammatory demyelinating polyneuropathy (CIDP) should be considered when faced with a chronic neuropathy with a non-length-dependent pattern of clinical deficits.

- The temporal evolution can also be characterized by the progression of symptoms: *progressive*, *relapsing*, or *monophasic*. In very broad terms, neuropathies with metabolic, toxic, nutritional, and genetically determined etiologies, as well as those that are idiopathic, tend to have a slowly progressive course unless the underlying condition is corrected. Relapsing neuropathies, especially those that are generalized or asymmetric, raise concern for a dysimmune or inflammatory process. A monophasic course is characteristic of GBS but can also be seen after toxin exposure and some presumed inflammatory conditions, such as diabetic lumbosacral radiculoplexopathy and neuralgic amyotrophy.

Descriptions of Polyneuropathies by Etiology

Length-Dependent Polyneuropathies

The most common polyneuropathy pattern is the length-dependent pattern (i.e., distal-predominant or stocking-glove). As this pattern first affects the longest nerves at their most distal segments, symptoms and signs are first recognized in the distal lower limbs. As the neuropathy progresses, shorter nerves become affected and clinical deficits can be appreciated in more proximal areas. The distal most segments of peripheral nerves may be particularly vulnerable to injury due to disrupted axonal transport and higher metabolic demand relative to more proximal segments.

With the important exception of CMT, sensory symptoms and signs usually predominate in length-dependent neuropathies; hence most patients present with negative and positive sensory symptoms and signs. Thus, the clinical presentation is of numbness, often accompanied by paresthesias, burning discomfort, and sensitivity to touch in the toes and feet in small fiber sensory-predominant neuropathies and gait imbalance in large fiber sensory-predominant neuropathies. Initial clinical findings are loss of sensation in the distal lower limbs, followed by loss of Achilles reflexes. In most length-dependent polyneuropathies, motor symptoms and signs develop later, with weakness of intrinsic foot muscles followed in turn by foot drop and weakness of intrinsic hand muscles. Electrophysiologic studies usually show reduced motor and sensory response amplitudes with preserved distal latencies and conduction velocities. As noted, CMT is unique in presenting with motor symptoms and, in CMT1, slow conduction velocities. In addition, several etiologies, usually those with prominent small fiber sensory symptoms, never progress to demonstrate significant motor involvement (Table 5.3).

The most common causes of length-dependent polyneuropathy fall into a small number of etiologic categories as follows:

- Metabolic disruption (e.g., diabetes mellitus or uremic neuropathy)
- Toxic exposure (e.g., alcohol or drug-induced)
- Hereditary (Charcot-Marie-Tooth)
- Vitamin deficiency (e.g., B12 deficiency, which causes a neuropathy in addition to subacute combined degeneration of the spinal cord)

About 30% of the time, despite an extensive investigation, the cause of length-dependent polyneuropathy remains unknown (idiopathic) [3] (Case 5.1).

Case 5.1
A 51-year-old woman presented with a 2–3-year history of foot pain. Symptoms began in the right second toe, and she saw a podiatrist at that time. Surgery for a presumed Morton's neuroma did not improve her symptoms, and they subsequently spread to involve all toes and the distal aspects of the feet. Symptoms have progressed gradually, and she now experiences burning discomfort and sharp, shooting

Table 5.3 Distinguishing features of several etiologies of acquired polyneuropathy

Etiology	Distinguishing neuropathic features
Associated with endocrinopathies	
Diabetes mellitus	Most commonly painful, sensory or sensorimotor, length-dependent distribution. Autonomic dysfunction sometimes occurs
Hypothyroid	Distal, painful, sensory. Weakness may be present due to a concurrent myopathy
Associated with systemic disease	
Connective tissue disease (rheumatoid arthritis, lupus, Sjogren's syndrome)	Usually length-dependent sensorimotor; may present with multiple mononeuropathies from vasculitis
Liver disease	Difficult to distinguish from neuropathy associated with other causes of liver damage (e.g., alcohol, viral hepatitis)
Renal failure	Usually length-dependent sensorimotor
Related to nutritional deficiency	
Vitamin deficiency (B12, B6)	Most commonly length-dependent, sensory-predominant. May have spastic paraparesis if corticospinal tract involvement (B12)
Copper	Similar to B12 deficiency (axonal sensorimotor neuropathy with corticospinal tract and dorsal column involvement)
Toxic	
Medications (common)	Most medications toxic to nerve produce axonal, length-dependent neuropathies
Alcohol	Length-dependent, sensory-predominant, large and small fiber
Heavy metals (exceedingly rare)	Lead, motor neuropathy with encephalopathy; mercury, ataxia, sensorimotor neuropathy, encephalopathy, GI symptoms Arsenic, painful sensorimotor neuropathy, abdominal discomfort, may resemble Guillain-Barré syndrome, Mees' lines on finger and toe nails

pains in the toes of both feet. She endorses possible reduction in tactile perception but no imbalance or falls. Pain is perceived as on the surface of the skin, and there is no aching discomfort. At times she finds bedsheets irritating and has to uncover her feet at night. Symptoms are most bothersome at night. They are less bothersome during the day, but she indicates that they tend to be worse after a busy day with a lot of standing and walking. Neuropathic pain questionnaire (NPQ) score is 0.37, indicating a likely neuropathic etiology. Past medical history is notable only for well-controlled hypertension and mild obesity (body mass index 33). Review of systems and family history are negative. She has about three glasses of wine weekly and denies known toxic exposures.

General physical examination is unremarkable. In particular there are no areas of tenderness in the feet, and there are no stigmata of vascular compromise. Neurologic examination demonstrates the following: mental status and cranial nerve examinations are normal. Extremity tone, bulk, and strength are normal. Perception of vibration and light touch are normal. Perception of pinprick is reduced distal to the ankles. Reflexes, including Achilles reflexes, are preserved. Coordination and gait are normal. Romberg sign is not present.

Normal or negative laboratory studies include complete blood count, vitamin B12 level, Sjogren's antibodies, sedimentation rate, and hepatitis C serology. A 2-h oral glucose tolerance test demonstrates a fasting glucose of 104 mg/dl, and a 2-h glucose of 159 mg/dl. Fasting triglyceride level is 307 mg/dl.

Nerve conduction studies are normal. Quantitative sensory testing demonstrates elevation of warm perception threshold in the foot. Epidermal nerve fiber density is reduced in the foot (3.3 ENF/mm) and normal in the calf (11.7 ENF/mm).

The patient is advised to manage signs of the metabolic syndrome with diet and exercise, and she chooses to begin swimming as it does not exacerbate weight-bearing on the feet. She treats her symptoms with 1% clonidine gel applied to the feet at night and 300 mg of gabapentin at bedtime. Over time her symptoms become more bothersome during the day, and, because she does not tolerate more frequent gabapentin dosing, she takes duloxetine 60 mg daily. With this combination of interventions, symptoms are tolerable and non-disabling.

Discussion: Small fiber neuropathy is a prevalent condition for which people often first seek care from podiatry. The presenting complaint is often positive sensory symptoms, but negative symptoms and signs are almost always present as well. Foot pain that is precipitated by weight-bearing and relieved when supine is most often musculoskeletal and not neuropathic, in which the converse occurs. The neuropathic pain questionnaire [4] and other discriminative instruments can be used to predict whether pain is neuropathic or non-neuropathic.

Proposed diagnostic criteria for small fiber neuropathy suggest that the diagnosis be made on the basis of presence of a combination of reduced sensation on examination, abnormal quantitative sensory testing (QST), and abnormal ENF density [5, 6]. Of course this leaves open the possibility that two psychophysical test results alone, without pathological or physiological confirmation, could be sufficient. We suggest that an objective measure such as ENF density or sudomotor testing be included.

Many cases of SFN have no recognized etiology. The metabolic syndrome may be disproportionately prevalent among people with SFN, although even this is a subject of controversy [7, 8]. Other recognized causes include HIV infection, chronic hepatitis C infection, often with cryoglobulinemia, Sjogren's syndrome, and antiretroviral drugs [9]. In idiopathic cases deficits typically progress slowly over a matter of years and do not significantly limit activities of daily living but can cause disabling pain. Medications with a strong evidence base for benefit in neuropathic pain management include duloxetine, pregabalin, gabapentin, and intermediate-dose tricyclic agents [10]. Although the evidence base for topical therapies is less extensive, they are often used initially if the area of pain is limited to avoid potential side effects of systemic agents.

Generally speaking, the treatment for acquired length-dependent axonal neuropathies is treatment of the underlying etiology. Supportive care is also essential. Pain and other positive sensory symptoms are managed with appropriate medications.

Gait instability and functional limitations are treated with physical and occupational therapy interventions. Orthotics can be helpful for some patients.

Charcot-Marie-Tooth

The hereditary neuropathies, often referred to as Charcot-Marie-Tooth (CMT), are a group of inherited disorders of nerve classified by pathology (axonal or demyelinating), mode of inheritance, and gene affected [11, 12].

Although the phenotype has some variability depending on the genotype, CMT is marked by variably severe weakness and atrophy in the feet, calves, and hands, hyporeflexia or areflexia, and distal-predominant sensory loss. In more severe cases, proximal weakness and even ventilatory dysfunction are seen. Unlike acquired length-dependent neuropathies, in CMT, motor signs and symptoms generally predominate (Fig. 5.1). Nerve conduction studies in CMT demonstrate either striking slowing of conduction, indicating a primary disorder of myelin (CMT1), or low amplitude responses with normal or near-normal conduction, indicating a primary axonal disorder (CMT2) (Table 5.4).

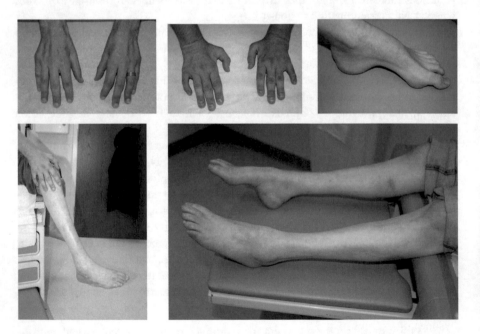

Fig. 5.1 Clinical features of Charcot-Marie-Tooth (CMT). Clockwise from top left: muscle atrophy in hand, foot, and calf

Table 5.4 The most common known forms of CMT. All noted are autosomal dominant except for CMT1X, which is X-linked

Designation	Gene
CMT1A	PMP22 duplication
CMT1B	MPZ
CMT2A	MFN2
CMT1X	GJB1
HNPP	PMP22 deletion

CMT1

CMT1 is the most common form of hereditary neuropathy and is caused by mutations of proteins that support myelin structure and function. Nerve conduction studies are characterized by slow nerve conduction velocities (<38 m/s in the median nerve; normal >48). Although nerve biopsy is now very rarely performed in cases of suspected CMT, reduction of myelinated nerve fibers and onion bulbs (indicating recurrent demyelination and remyelination) are seen on nerve biopsy in CMT1. The most common form of CMT1 is due to a duplication in the PMP22 gene (CMT1A) [13]. Note that deletion of the PMP22 gene causes a different phenotype (HNPP). Patients with CMT1A usually present in the first decade of life with ankle sprains, foot dorsiflexion weakness, and distal numbness. Symptoms and signs progress gradually throughout life.

Case 5.2
A 53 year old man was seen in follow-up for progressive limb weakness and disability. His earliest recollection of his condition is of recurrent ankle sprains when running or participating in sports in childhood. At age 16 he underwent surgery for pes cavus, hammertoe deformity, and varus deformity at the ankles. Surgery initially appeared to help, but in subsequent years he developed increasing pain at the right ankle. In adult life he developed increasing weakness at the ankles, with frequent falls due to tripping or losing balance when standing. Ankle foot orthoses helped with these, but he had great difficulty finding a pair that he could wear without discomfort from pressure. Past medical history is otherwise unremarkable. Family history is notable for similar symptoms among his father, two paternal aunts, three cousins, and his one son.

In recent years, he has required the use of a walker because of instability and weakness in the lower limbs. He tires easily and in the evening often has to ascend the stairs to his second floor bedroom on his knees. He previously worked as a machinist but applied for Social Security disability after his employer indicated that he was no longer able to keep up with the pace at work and expressed concern about his safety in the workplace. His chief complaints now are right hip pain, fatigue, dyspnea on exertion, and difficulty with activities of daily living because of loss of fine motor control. He would also like to know if he can continue driving, as he has found it increasingly difficult to drive long distances because of lower limb sensory loss, weakness, and fatigue. Further questioning regarding fatigue reveals a report of frequent nocturnal awakenings and non-restorative sleep.

General physical examination demonstrates a moderately obese individual (BMI 31.6). There is tenderness at the right sacroiliac joint that reproduces his reported hip pain. Examination of the extremities demonstrates venous stasis changes and symmetric mild to moderate edema in the feet and ankles. There are large callouses laterally on both feet but no skin breakdown. Pedal pulses are 2+. There are multiple well-healed surgical scars in the feet and ankles, deformities at the ankle joints, and pes planus.

Neurologic examination demonstrates the following: mental status and cranial nerve examinations are normal. Sensory examination demonstrates reduced perception of touch and pin distal to the knees in the lower limbs and the proximal interphalangeal joints of both hands. Vibration perception is absent in the lower limbs and mildly reduced in the hands. He is areflexic. Motor examination demonstrates marked symmetric atrophy in the forearms, intrinsic hand muscles, calves, and feet. Manual muscle testing demonstrates the following symmetric findings on an MRC scale: shoulder abduction 5, elbow flexion 4+, elbow extension 4-, wrist extension 3, wrist flexion 4, interossei 1, and thumb abduction 2. In the lower limbs, hip flexion strength is 5, hip extension is 5, knee extension is 5, knee flexion is 4-, ankle dorsiflexion is 0, and ankle plantar flexion is estimated at 3. He walks using his walker, with both steppage and Trendelenburg components. He hyperextends at the knee joints when standing.

Motor conduction studies demonstrate absent sensory potentials throughout, absent compound muscle action potentials in the lower limbs, and moderate attenuation of compound muscle action potentials in the upper limbs. Upper extremity motor conduction velocities are in the 11–16 m/s in all segments of all nerves tested, without focal motor conduction block or abnormal temporal dispersion.

Discussion: This patient has a moderately severe CMT1 phenotype. The most common cause is a PMP22 duplication or CMT1, and genetic testing should begin with testing for this. Note that he has substantial functional concerns including the following:

- Impairment of ADLs, IADLs, mobility, and balance due to weakness of distal upper limbs as well as proximal and distal lower limbs.
- Foot pain due to a combination of factors including ankle instability, foot deformity, ankle swelling, and ill-fitting ankle-foot orthoses.
- Fatigue, likely due to excessive work required in walking and other daily tasks, pain, and sleep-disordered breathing. This may be exacerbated by weakness of the ventilatory muscles, which can occur in moderately severe CMT phenotypes.
- Musculoskeletal pain – this is extremely common in people with moderately severe weakness and gait disturbances from CMT.
- Concerns about driving.

Evaluation and management of these complex problems should include the following:

- Occupational and physical therapy evaluations for help with IADLs, mobility, and balance.
- Physical therapy, orthopedic, or pain medicine evaluation for sacroiliac joint pain. The patient may benefit from stretching, pool therapy, and interventional approaches.
- Orthotics, podiatry, and possibly foot and ankle surgery evaluations.
- Pulmonary function studies with seated and supine testing.
- Sleep medicine consultation with possible polysomnography.
- Driver's evaluation. The patient may benefit from hand controls.

CMT2

In most cases CMT2 is caused by protein mutations that support axon structure and function. Nerve conduction studies are characterized by normal or near-normal nerve conduction velocities (median motor conduction velocity > 38 m/s) with reduced motor and sensory response amplitudes. Histologic features include reduction of myelinated nerve fibers without prominent onion bulbs.

Other Forms of CMT

CMT1 and CMT2 are the most prevalent forms of CMT. Dominant intermediate CMT (DI-CMT) designates forms with intermediate conduction velocities. CMT4 designates autosomal recessive forms. Distal hereditary motor neuropathy (dHMN) is a genetically determined pure motor syndrome that is typically classified as CMT. Numerous mutations have been identified as causes of each form [14].

Regardless of the primary pathology, disability in CMT develops because of progressive loss of axons. Thus, patients with CMT1 demonstrate very slow nerve conduction velocity throughout life but develop disability gradually over several decades as axons degenerate. This illustrates two important points: first, conduction slowing alone does not cause weakness or numbness. Clinical dysfunction due to disorders of myelin is due either to secondary axon loss (as occurs in CMT1) or conduction block (block of the wave of depolarization due to focal demyelination, as occurs in CIDP (see below). Second, genetic disorders of myelin lead to axon loss, indicating that normal myelin plays a role in maintaining axonal integrity.

Generalized (Non-Length-Dependent) Polyneuropathies

Non-length-dependent polyneuropathies can affect both proximal and distal nerve segments. With the important exception of multifocal motor neuropathy, discussed below, both motor and sensory fibers are affected, and deep tendon reflexes may be reduced or absent in both proximal and distal areas [3]. Unlike the length-dependent pattern in which the fundamental pathophysiologic insult is usually that of axonal degeneration, the most common non-length-dependent polyneuropathies, chronic inflammatory demyelinating polyneuropathy (CIDP) and Guillain-Barré syndrome (GBS), usually reflect demyelinating pathophysiology.

Chronic Inflammatory Demyelinating Polyneuropathy (CIDP)

Typical CIDP

Typical CIDP is an immune-mediated non-length-dependent polyneuropathy [15]. Affected individuals develop bilateral proximal and distal weakness and sensory loss. Deep tendon reflexes are reduced or absent. Unlike GBS, in which disease activity reaches a nadir by 4 weeks, in CIDP active immune dysfunction is defined as continuing for a minimum of 8 weeks. The course may be monophasic, chronic relapsing, stepwise progressive, or steady progressive (Table 5.5). Nerve

Table 5.5 Clinical diagnostic CIDP criteria according to EFNS/PNS 2010

(1). Inclusion criteria
(a) Typical CIDP
• Chronically progressive, stepwise, or recurrent symmetric proximal and distal weakness and sensory dysfunction of all extremities, developing over at least 2 months; cranial nerves may be affected
• Absent or reduced tendon reflexes in all extremities
(b) Atypical CIDP (still considered CIDP but with different features)
• Predominantly distal (distal acquired demyelinating symmetric, DADS)
• Asymmetric [multifocal acquired demyelinating sensory and motor neuropathy (MADSAM), Lewis-Sumner syndrome]
• Focal (e.g., involvement of the brachial or lumbosacral plexus or of one or more peripheral nerves in one upper or lower limb)
• Pure motor
• Pure sensory (including chronic immune sensory polyradiculopathy affecting the central process of the primary sensory neuron)
(2). Exclusion criteria
• *Borrelia burgdorferi* infection (Lyme disease), diphtheria, drug or toxin exposure probably to have caused the neuropathy
• Hereditary demyelinating neuropathy
• Prominent sphincter disturbance
• Diagnosis of multifocal motor neuropathy
• IgM monoclonal gammopathy with high titer antibodies to myelin-associated glycoprotein
• Other causes for a demyelinating neuropathy including POEMS syndrome, osteosclerotic myeloma, diabetic and nondiabetic lumbosacral radiculoplexus neuropathy. PNS lymphoma and amyloidosis may occasionally have demyelinating features

With permission John Wiley and Sons © 2010 [16]

conduction studies show characteristic electrophysiologic evidence of demyelination, including motor conduction slowing, conduction block, temporal dispersion, distal latency prolongation, and F wave prolongation. Cerebrospinal fluid classically shows elevated CSF protein with no mononuclear cells (albuminocytologic dissociation). Nerve biopsy, although rarely performed for diagnosis, may identify evidence of segmental demyelination and remyelination, loss of myelinated fibers, occasional onion bulb formation, and occasional inflammatory infiltration into interstitial and perivascular areas.

The pathologic process in CIDP is dysimmune, T-cell, and macrophage-mediated demyelination. Although the clinical presentation is notable for widespread and often symmetric findings, the pathological process is nonuniform, affecting myelinated axons in a patchy distribution. Regardless of the site of demyelination along the course of an axon, the physiologic outcome is the same: conduction block or inability to conduct an action potential along the full length of the axon. The clinical outcome, in turn, is a sensory or motor deficit in the distribution affected. CIDP is generally not part of a multisystem immune disorder; hence, routine inflammatory markers in blood are negative, and other organs are unaffected.

First-line treatment for CIDP is either corticosteroids or intravenous immunoglubulin (IVIg) [15]. Regardless of which is used, tapering should be attempted upon normalization of strength or a plateau in improvement. Plasmapheresis (PLEX) is also an effective treatment option but is typically reserved for patients' refractory to corticosteroids and IVIg because it is more cumbersome to administer. In some patients an additional immunomodulating agent such as azathioprine, mycophenolate mofetil, cyclophosphamide, or cyclosporine may be used, but none have been proven in high-quality randomized controlled trials to be beneficial in CIDP [17]. These agents are often used in an effort to facilitate tapering of corticosteroids, and their use must be considered on an individual basis (Case 5.3).

Case 5.3

A 58-year-old woman with an otherwise unremarkable past medical history presented with numbness and paresthesias bilaterally in her feet and hands. Symptoms are symmetric, and onset in the hands and feet was simultaneous. Over several months, the intensity of her symptoms slowly worsened, and within 3 months of symptom onset, she developed weakness in her hands and legs. She was having trouble turning keys in a lock and occasionally tripped while walking. Five months after symptoms began, standing from the floor became difficult.

Examination at that time revealed bilateral and symmetric weakness in her proximal and distal lower limbs and distal upper limbs, reduced vibration perception in the feet and toes, and diffusely reduced or absent deep tendon reflexes. Nerve conduction studies revealed preserved motor response amplitudes but patchy conduction slowing. Specifically, in two motor nerve segments slowing was only minor, but in three nerve segments, motor conduction velocities were <70% of the lower limit of normal, indicating evidence of demyelination as the primary process. Conduction block was also seen in the median nerve in the forearm. CSF protein was 98 mg/dL, with 0 white blood cells (albuminocytologic dissociation). Serum protein immunofixation was normal.

The patient was diagnosed with CIDP and treated with IVIg 2 gm/kg loading divided over 3 days followed by 1 gm/kg maintenance every 3 weeks. Symptoms began to improve within 5 days of initiating treatment. Three months after treatment initiation, her strength was normal. She reported mild residual numbness and paresthesias in the distal lower and upper limbs but otherwise was able to perform most of her usual daily activities without difficulty. Over the following months, IVIg was tapered by extending the treatment interval by 1 week every infusion cycle. When the treatment interval reached 5 weeks, she noticed return of numbness and weakness similar to when her disease began.

Discussion: This patient's symptoms and signs, electrophysiology, and CSF profile are classic for "typical" CIDP. Note the proximal and distal symptoms and early involvement of the upper limbs. She was treated with evidence-based IVIg dosing: 2 gm/kg loading followed by 1 gm/kg every 3 weeks [18, 19]. One of the challenges with maintenance treatment in patients with CIDP is finding the "best" dose for each patient. One approach is to start with an evidence-based dosing regimen as was done here. Once maximum improvement and stability are achieved, the treatment interval is gradually extended. If a well-documented relapse occurs, the dosing interval can be set at the longest interval that provides clinical stability, in this case every 4–5 weeks. Thereafter, if the patient does well, the treatment dose can be tapered as tolerated.

Atypical CIDP

Not all patients with CIDP present with "typical" clinical features. Variants of CIDP that are still classified under the CIDP umbrella but which have different symptoms and signs include sensory CIDP, motor CIDP, Lewis Sumner syndrome, and DADS. Sensory CIDP and motor CIDP are characterized by non-length dependent sensory or motor syndromes. Those with sensory CIDP often have sensory ataxia and reduced reflexes. Patients with motor CIDP have generalized weakness not limited to individual named nerve distributions, and importantly are without upper motor neuron signs. Lewis Sumner Syndrome is an asymmetric variant of CIDP and will be discussed further in the multifocal polyneuropathy section. Distal acquired demyelinating sensory (DADS) neuropathy is a CIDP variant which is distal-predominant but not length-dependent. Affected patients experience slowly progressive, symmetric, distally accentuated large fiber-type sensory symptoms [20]. Specifically, people with DADS neuropathy develop imbalance due to sensory loss ("sensory ataxia"), loss of joint position, and a Romberg sign from large fiber sensory loss. Reflexes are reduced or absent. Weakness, if present, is isolated distally. Although the most prominent symptoms are sensory, nerve conduction studies show characteristic demyelinating change in distal segments of motor nerves. A monoclonal protein (usually IgM) is detected in up to two thirds of patients, and up to two

Table 5.6 Variants of Guillain-Barré syndrome

1. Acute inflammatory demyelinating polyneuropathy (AIDP)
2. Acute motor axonal neuropathy (AMAN)
3. Acute motor-sensory axonal neuropathy (AMSAN)
4. Miller Fisher syndrome (MFS)

thirds of these have detectable serum antibodies to myelin- associated glycoprotein (MAG). MAG is an adhesion protein in compact myelin, and biopsies of nerve in affected individuals demonstrate decompaction of myelin [21]. Patients with DADS and MAG antibodies generally have a more indolent course than patients with typical CIDP but also have a poorer response to immunomodulatory therapy. For these reasons, anti-MAG antibody associated neuropathy is not classified as a variant of CIDP but instead is considered to be a distinct disorder.

Guillain-Barré Syndrome (GBS)

GBS is a diffuse polyradiculoneuropathy which develops over days or weeks, reaching its nadir (greatest severity) 2–4 weeks after onset. Classically GBS presents as symmetric proximal and distal weakness with reduced or absent reflexes. Severity ranges from minimal disability with maintenance of gait to complete quadriparesis and respiratory failure requiring mechanical ventilation. GBS is usually accompanied by positive sensory symptoms but relatively modest sensory deficits. There is often striking autonomic involvement, leading to a resting tachycardia and fluctuations in blood pressure. The condition is preceded by infection in 65% of cases, usually upper respiratory tract infection or gastroenteritis, which is consistent with the view that it is of autoimmune etiology and is sometimes triggered by an immune attack upon a foreign antigen which shares an epitope with a component of peripheral nerve. Several subtypes or variants of GBS have been recognized [22]. Subtypes may be categorized by the modality affected (pure motor or pure sensory) or pathophysiology (axonal or demyelinating) (Table 5.6).

Acute Inflammatory Demyelinating Polyneuropathy (AIDP)

AIDP is the most common form of GBS in western populations. Symptoms and signs are both proximal and distal and evolve over days to up to 4 weeks. Facial weakness, ophthalmoplegia, back pain, autonomic dysfunction, and respiratory failure may also occur. Recognition of autonomic instability and respiratory distress is of critical importance, as these can be fatal. Between 20 and 30% of patients develop respiratory failure and require mechanical ventilation [23].

Neuromuscular examination in AIDP demonstrates motor-predominant deficits in a generalized pattern, often with facial weakness, and reduced or absent reflexes. Cerebrospinal fluid classically shows albuminocytologic disassociation.

Nerve conduction studies may reveal evidence of demyelination including prolonged or absent F waves (often the earliest abnormality), conduction velocity slowing, conduction block, and temporal dispersion. Although CSF and nerve conduction studies are important diagnostic tests, these abnormalities may take 2 weeks or more to develop and so may be normal in the hyperacute stage.

Rapid initiation of treatment is crucial [24]. Plasma exchange (PLEX) (200–250 mL/kg total exchange volume divided over 10–14 days) and IVIg (2 gm/kg divided over 5 days) have both been shown to be effective. Early treatment within 7–10 days is best. The decision whether to use PLEX or IVIg is dependent upon availability and relative medical contraindications. Supportive care is equally important. Supportive care includes frequent respiratory and cardiac monitoring, deep vein thrombosis prophylaxis, pain control, physical therapy, infection prevention (sepsis, pneumonia), and nutritional support.

AIDP is a monophasic illness that usually reaches a nadir by 4 weeks with recovery over months to about 2 years. Residual deficits are common. Indicators of a poor prognosis include age greater than 60 years, abrupt onset of severe weakness, need for mechanical ventilation, and early reduction in compound muscle action potential amplitudes [25]. Even with rapid treatment and aggressive supportive care, mortality is 5% (Case 5.4).

Case 5.4

A 49-year-old man presented to an outpatient clinic appointment for evaluation of upper extremity weakness. His past medical history was remarkable only for a similar episode of evolving upper limb weakness 17 years prior that reached nadir within 3 weeks and recovered without any residual motor or sensory deficits. He was entirely normal until the current episode, which followed an upper respiratory tract infection by about 2 weeks. At initial presentation, he reported proximal symmetric weakness in his upper limbs that had worsened over about 4 days. He denied sensory symptoms other than new achy pain in his neck and mid-back. He denied lower limb weakness. Neurologic examination disclosed 3/5 proximal upper limb weakness, 4/5 distal upper limb weakness, and hyporeflexia in the upper limbs. Cranial nerve examination, lower limb strength, and sensory examination were normal.

Nerve conduction studies (Table 5.7) revealed normal motor and sensory conduction studies but prolonged median and ulnar minimum F wave latencies. Needle electromyography demonstrated reduced recruitment in clinically weak upper limb muscles. The patient was immediately admitted to the hospital for further evaluation and treatment.

CSF analysis upon admission showed one white blood cell and a protein of 52 mg/dL. IVIg 2 gm/kg divided over 5 days was started for a clinical suspicion of GBS. Over the following 3 days, he deteriorated. On day 3 of admission, examination revealed moderately severe and symmetric weakness as follows: proximal upper limbs were 2/5, distal upper limbs 3/5, proximal lower limbs 4/5, and distal lower limbs 3/5. Deep tendon reflexes were absent. Sensory deficits to vibration were detected in his hands and feet. He was able to ambulate with assistance. Cranial

Table 5.7 Nerve conduction studies performed 4 days after symptom onset

Sensory NCS			
Nerve/site	Rec. Site	CV (m/s)	Amplitude (uV)
L median – Dig II			
Wrist	Dig II	54.9	30.8
R median – Dig II			
Wrist	Dig II	58.4	23.1
L ulnar – Dig V			
Wrist	Dig V	54.5	17.3
R ulnar – Dig V			
Wrist	Dig V	50.1	16.2
L sural – Lat mall			
Calf	Ankle	44.2	21.9

Motor NCS					
Nerve/site	Rec. Site	Latency (ms)	Amplitude (mV)	Duration (ms)	CV (m/s)
L median – APB					
Wrist	APB	4.22	13.0	5.9	
Elbow	APB	9.06	11.9	6.1	54.5
R median – APB					
Wrist	APB	3.68	8.8	5.2	
Elbow	APB	8.31	8.7	5.5	56.1
L ulnar – ADM					
Wrist	ADM	3.61	8.6	5.3	
B elbow	ADM	7.04	8.2	5.9	60.3
A elbow	ADM	9.55	7.7	6.2	55.5
R ulnar – ADM					
Wrist	ADM	3.49	9.1	5.5	
B elbow	ADM	8.2	8.2	5.9	59.8
A elbow	ADM	9.38	7.7	6.0	56.9
L peroneal – EDB					
Ankle	EDB	5.26	6.1	5.3	
Fib head	EDB	12.24	6.1	5.4	45.3
Pop fossa	EDB	14.11	6.0	5.4	53.0
L tibial – AH					
Ankle	AH	5.78	8.2	5.1	
Knee	AH	15.83	6.8	5.9	46.8

F wave	
Nerve	Min F latency (ms)
L median	35.5
R median	37.2
L ulnar	38.9
R ulnar	33.8
L tibial	57.1

Table 5.8 Nerve conduction studies performed 3 weeks after symptom onset

Sensory NCS			
Nerve/site	Rec. Site	CV (m/s)	Amplitude (uV)
L median – Dig II			
Wrist	Dig II	54.9	20.3
L ulnar – Dig V			
Wrist	Dig V	52.2	12.3
L sural – Lat mall			
Calf	Ankle	44.1	7.4

Motor NCS					
Nerve/site	Rec. Site	Latency (ms)	Amplitude (mV)	Duration (ms)	CV (m/s)
L median – APB					
Wrist	APB	5.99	3.4	9.11	
Elbow	APB	11.04	0.7	12.6	45.5
L ulnar – ADM					
Wrist	ADM	5.94	4.7	6.61	
B elbow	ADM	12.10	3.2	7.76	37.2
A elbow	ADM	14.69	2.6	7.66	47.0
L peroneal – EDB					
Ankle	EDB	5.31	2.0	8.75	
Fib head	EDB	14.69	0.4	9.69	35.5
Pop fossa	EDB	17.92	0.4	15.52	34.1
L tibial – AH					
Ankle	AH	7.58	2.2	7.86	
Knee	AH	17.83	1.1	7.96	37.3

F wave	
Nerve	Min F latency (ms)
L median	44.43
L ulnar	53.59
L tibial	61.09

nerve examination remained normal. IVIg was completed on day 5 of admission. His condition remained unchanged for 1 week, followed by modest improvement.

Approximately 3 weeks after his initial hospitalization (10 days after IVIg completion), he worsened again. He lost the ability to ambulate and was unable perform any meaningful activities with his upper limbs. He developed shortness of breath, but FVC remained above 70% of the predicted value, and NIF remained between -40 and -60 cm H_2O. Mechanical ventilation was not needed, and at no time during his hospital course did he develop facial weakness, diplopia, dysarthria, dysphagia, or autonomic instability. Repeat nerve conduction studies (Table 5.8) now showed reduced motor amplitudes in the upper and lower limbs. Variable degrees of distal motor latency prolongation, conduction block, and conduction velocity slowing were identified in the median, ulnar, tibial, and peroneal motor nerves.

He was treated with another course of IVIg 2 gm/kg again divided over 5 days. Upon completion of the second course of IVIg, strength began to improve. He was able to stand with assistance and regained some meaningful arm movements. Within 2 weeks he could stand independently, and within 3 weeks he could ambulate with a walker. At 3 months from nadir, he could walk without any support. Climbing stairs remained difficult and he still could not run. Arm strength improved more slowly, but he was now able to dress himself, use a keyboard, and feed himself. No further deterioration occurred after the second course of IVIg.

Discussion: While GBS is usually monophasic condition that reaches nadir within 4 weeks, recurrences have been reported in about 5% of patients. As was the case in this patient, recurrent symptoms are often similar to prior episodes, but clinical severity can be variable. In both of this patient's episodes, upper limb weakness was the first and most severely affected deficit. Although GBS is typically described as an "ascending" paralysis, upper limb, oropharyngeal, or respiratory weakness may begin with or before the onset of lower extremity weakness. Furthermore when weakness does begin in the lower extremities, it often begins as proximal weakness. This reflects the fact that GBS is a polyradiculoneuropathy, with prominent involvement of nerve roots (hence with elevated CSF protein), in contradistinction to a length-dependent polyneuropathy, in which nerve roots are unaffected and symptoms always begin distally. A more distinguishing clinical feature of GBS than ascending progression of paralysis is the presence of rapidly worsening proximal and distal motor and/or sensory symptoms, which are relatively symmetric in distribution [22–25].

It is also important to recognize that nerve conduction studies and CSF may be normal or only mildly abnormal early in the disease course. While CSF classically demonstrates elevated protein with normal cell count (cytoalbuminologic dissociation), this is found in less than half of patients when tested very early in the disease course. Only after a week does CSF sensitivity reach 80%. The diagnostic value of CSF resides more in absence of pleocytosis than the presence of cytoalbuminologic dissociation. If more than 50 white cells/μl are present, the diagnosis of GBS should be strongly reconsidered, with attention turning to GBS mimics that include HIV, Lyme disease, sarcoid, and lymphoma. NCS also may require several weeks before the characteristic demyelinating features of distal latency prolongation, conduction block, temporal dispersion, and conduction velocity slowing are maximally appreciated. Within the first week, absent or prolonged H-reflexes or F wave responses may be the only abnormality, and in up to 13% of cases, the initial study is normal [22–25]. Needle EMG can be helpful to differentiate very early GBS from other causes of acute or subacute symmetric proximal weakness such as myopathy. GBS typically shows rapidly firing but normal-appearing motor units with reduced recruitment in clinically weak muscles, as opposed to an early recruitment pattern, often with short-duration motor units that is characteristic of myopathy.

This case also calls attention to treatment challenges that are sometimes encountered. About 10% of GBS patients treated with IVIg or plasma exchange deteriorate after initial improvement or stabilization (sometimes referred to as treatment-related fluctuations). If such fluctuations occur within 8 weeks of disease onset, they may represent a monophasic but prolonged immune response with ongoing inflammation and nerve injury. Currently there is no convincing evidence that re-treating with

IVIg or plasma exchange provides patients with extra benefit. However, it has been shown that GBS patients that have a low increase of serum IgG levels after a standard IVIg dose have slower recovery and worse prognosis compared to those with larger increases in serum IgG. The reasons for this are unknown but may be due to individual variability in IgG catabolism or more directly related to the severity or breadth of the immune-mediated nerve damage. Most would agree that if a patient fails to respond to first-line therapy or if treatment-related fluctuations develop after initial treatment, re-treatment with IVIg or PE is reasonable. The SID-GBS trial (second IVIg dose in GBS patients) will provide insight on the role of repeat IVIg treatment in GBS patients with poor prognosis [26].

Acute Motor Axonal Neuropathy (AMAN)

AMAN is the most common GBS variant in China. Antecedent illness occurs in 30–85% and is most commonly *C. jejuni* infection [27]. AMAN is believed to be caused by immune-mediated attack on the nodal axolemma, and molecular mimicry of human gangliosides by *Campylobacter jejuni* lipo-oligosaccharides appears to play a key pathogenic role in post-*Campylobacter* cases. GM1 or Gd1a antibodies are present in many patients with AMAN [28]. Autoantibodies that bind to GM1 or GD1a gangliosides at the nodes of Ranvier may activate complement and lead to sodium channel damage [29]. Nerve conduction studies usually show normal sensory responses but reduced distal motor response amplitudes. Not uncommonly conduction block is also appreciated. While conduction block is usually taken as evidence of segmental demyelination, in AMAN it is caused by sodium channel dysfunction at the nodes of Ranvier. Patients experience rapidly progressive generalized weakness similar to AIDP but without sensory involvement. CSF findings are similar to AIDP. The therapeutic approach is also similar to AIDP.

Acute Motor-Sensory Axonal Neuropathy (AMSAN)

Like AIDP, patients with AMSAN experience acute or hyperacute onset of generalized motor and sensory deficits. Symptoms usually develop even faster than typical AIDP. Nerve conduction studies show low amplitude motor and sensory responses without evidence of demyelination. CSF may reveal albuminocytologic dissociation. Treatment is similar to AIDP. Prognosis is generally less favorable than AIDP and AMAN.

Miller Fisher Syndrome (MFS)

Classic MFS presents with a triad of ataxia, areflexia, and ophthalmoplegia [30]. Mild proximal weakness may also develop. CSF protein can be normal or elevated. Nerve conduction studies may show small sensory amplitudes without demyelinating features.

Motor responses are usually normal. MFS is associated with the presence of serum antibodies to GQ1b ganglioside in nearly all cases. Although IVIg may hasten MFS recovery, even without treatment MFS prognosis is generally good. Most patients return to full function in 3–5 months.

Sensory Ganglionopathy

Special note is also made of disorders that selectively affect the dorsal root ganglia. Affected patients developed proximal and distal sensory symptoms and signs but with spared motor function [31]. Early gait impairment due to proprioceptive loss (sensory ataxia) is common. Nerve conduction studies typically show reduced or absent sensory responses often in a non-length-dependent pattern. Motor responses and F waves are normal, but H-reflexes may be absent or delayed (Case 5.5).

Case 5.5
A 51-year-old woman was referred for electrodiagnostic evaluation of possible carpal tunnel syndrome because of a 10-year history of progressive sensory loss in the left hand. Nerve conduction studies demonstrated absent median and ulnar sensory nerve action potentials and normal motor conduction studies and electromyography. The study was interpreted as demonstrating a sensory neuropathy, and she was referred for neuromuscular consultation.

General medical history was notable only for vitiligo. Review of systems was notable for dry eyes and mouth, frequent dental caries, and aching in the lower limbs. She denied fever, night sweats, or weight loss and denied hematuria, hematochezia, or abnormal vaginal bleeding. Mammograms and Pap smears were up to date and negative, but she was due for a colonoscopy. General medical examination was normal.

Neurologic examination demonstrated the following: mental status and cranial nerve examinations were normal. Perception of light touch, pin, and vibration were reduced in the left hand diffusely, not respecting peripheral nerve territories. Vibration perception was mildly reduced in the toes. Motor examination demonstrated normal tone, bulk, and strength, although she had difficulty sustaining resistance in the intrinsic hand muscles on examination ("giveaway"). Bilateral biceps, patellar, and Achilles reflexes were absent. Coordination testing revealed pseudoathetosis in the left hand. Gait was normal. She swayed but did not fall on Romberg testing.

Laboratory testing demonstrated a positive SS-A antibody and negative SS-B, ANA, antineuronal nuclear, hepatitis C, Lyme, and tissue transglutaminase antibodies. Sedimentation rate, complement levels, ANCA, cryoglobulin, and vitamin B12 level were normal. A Schirmer's test confirmed reduced tear production. Chest X-ray was normal.

She was seen in rheumatology consultation and was given a diagnosis of Sjogren's syndrome based upon the presence of appropriate symptoms, confirmation of reduced tear production, and antibody positivity. She was placed on Plaquenil,

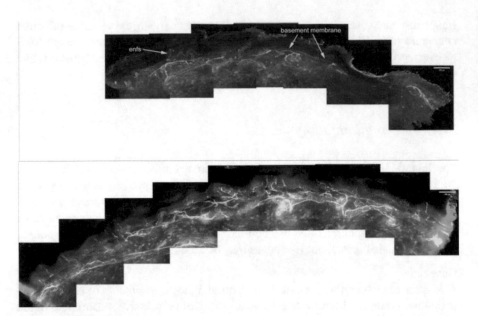

Fig. 5.2 Near-complete absence of epidermal nerve fibers (ENFs) in the calf with relative sparing of ENFs in the foot, demonstrating a small fiber neuropathy in a non-length dependent pattern. This pattern should raise suspicion of sensory ganglionopathy. Top: Calf image. Bottom: Foot image. enfs: epidermal nerve fibers (green); collagen in basement membrane and blood vessels in red. Montage courtesy of laboratory of William R Kennedy, M.D.

with some improvement in her lower limb aching. Neurologic follow-up over the subsequent 5 years demonstrated only minimal progression of functional deficits in the left hand and sensory loss in the feet (Fig. 5.2).

Discussion: Sensory ganglionopathy is most commonly a non-length-dependent process, with large and sometimes small fiber sensory symptoms and signs. The differential diagnosis of non-length dependent sensory loss in adolescents and adults includes platinum-based drug exposure (cisplatin, carboplatin, and oxaliplatin), para-neoplastic (often associated with anti-Hu or anti-CV2/CRMP-5 antibodies), and rarely vitamin B6 toxicity [31]. Sensory- predominant presentations of CIDP are usually distinguishable on the basis of nerve conduction studies but can be confused for ganglionopathy because phase cancellation commonly causes reduced sensory nerve action potential amplitude, rather than conduction slowing, in acquired demyelinating conditions. One variant of CIDP, chronic immune sensory polyradiculopathy (CISP) can be particularity challenging as the site of immune attack is at the dorsal nerve root [32]. Because the pathology is proximal to the dorsal root ganglion, sensory nerve conduction studies are typically normal. Idiopathic sensory ganglionopathy is a diagnosis of exclusion and may have a presumed autoimmune pathophysiology in some cases. In otherwise healthy adults that develop a sensory ganglionopathy it is important to explore the possibility of connective tissue disorders, and in particular Sjogren's syndrome.

Ganglionopathy in Sjogren's syndrome is often an indolent process, but immunotherapy might be justified in the context of acute deterioration. Appropriate management includes application of relevant therapies to assist with ADLs and fall prevention.

Multifocal Polyneuropathy

A polyneuropathy affecting multiple individual named nerves is referred to as a multifocal polyneuropathy or mononeuropathy multiplex. Mononeuropathy multiplex affects both sensory and motor components of individual named nerves and can affect cranial nerves as well. Symptoms often develop in a stepwise fashion and a subacute time course. Vasculitis and infiltration of peripheral nerve are the most notable causes of axonal mononeuropathy multiplex, while multifocal motor neuropathy (MMN) and Lewis-Sumner syndrome are the most common multifocal demyelinating conditions.

Vasculitis

Vasculitis can be isolated to the peripheral nervous system or associated with a systemic vasculitic condition (e.g., polyarteritis nodosa, Wegener's granulomatosis, or Churg-Strauss syndrome) or a connective tissue disorder (e.g., lupus or rheumatoid arthritis) [33]. Vasculitis can also be due to immune activation from chronic hepatitis C or HIV. In the case of HCV, cryoglobulins are often detectable in serum as well [34].

Vasculitis is an immune-mediated disorder directed against blood vessels. Transmural inflammatory cell infiltration and vessel wall necrosis results in peripheral nerve ischemia and infarction. Patients often develop acute onset of pain, weakness, and sensory loss in a named nerve distribution. Critically important in the evaluation of peripheral nerve vasculitis is investigation for an underlying systemic condition. Nerve conduction studies demonstrate the axonal nature of the process and can characterize the distribution and severity of nerve lesions. Nerve biopsy may be helpful to show the inflammatory process. The mainstay of treatment is usually prompt and aggressive immunosuppression, beginning with high-dose corticosteroids but often requiring concomitant treatment with cyclophosphamide or other agents (Case 5.6).

Case 5.6

A 37-year-old woman with a 6-month history of recurrent sinusitis developed burning pain in the left axilla radiating to the lateral aspect of the hand. Three weeks later, she developed right lower extremity pain and ankle dorsiflexion weakness. Over the course of the subsequent 2 months, pain and weakness progressed to the right upper limb and left foot, and she developed numbness on the right side of the face.

General medical systems review was notable for occasional exertional dyspnea, sinus "stuffiness," and unexplained 10-pound weight loss. The patient denied fever, night sweats, rash, joint pain, nausea, abdominal or pelvic pain, hematuria, hematochezia, or abnormal vaginal bleeding. Past medical history was unremarkable.

General physical examination was notable only for nasal polyps and subtle wheezes at the right lung base. Neurologic examination demonstrated the following: mental state and cranial nerve examinations were normal aside from dysesthesias to pinprick on the right side of the face. Sensation was diminished to light touch over the left lateral forearm, medial right hand, and both feet below the ankles, and vibration perception was absent in the toes and malleoli. Motor examination demonstrated atrophy in the right hand involving ulnar-innervated muscles only and the right anterior tibial compartment of the calf. Tone was reduced at the right ankle. Manual muscle testing demonstrated 4/5 strength in the interosseous muscles of the right hand, 4/5 strength of left ankle dorsiflexion, and 3/5 strength of right ankle dorsiflexion. Reflexes were absent at the left biceps and bilateral Achilles. Coordination was normal. She walked independently with a steppage gait.

Laboratory testing was notable for eosinophilia, marked elevation of sedimentation rate, CRP, and p-ANCA. Urinalysis demonstrated trace proteinuria and microscopic hematuria. Chest X-ray demonstrated several small hazy infiltrates. CT scan of chest abdomen and pelvis demonstrated patchy pulmonary infiltrates and was otherwise negative.

Nerve conduction studies demonstrated evidence of a multifocal sensory and motor axonal polyneuropathy; notably, the ulnar compound muscle action potential amplitude was normal on the left and attenuated on the right, and the peroneal compound muscle action potential amplitudes were attenuated on the left and absent on the right. No conduction velocity slowing was present in proximal nerve segments.

Sural nerve biopsy demonstrated perivascular inflammatory infiltrates with transmural inflammation of epineurial vessels and axon loss that was variable in severity within and between nerve fascicles (Fig. 5.3).

Rheumatology consultation was obtained. A diagnosis of eosinophilic granulomatosis with polyangiitis (Churg-Strauss syndrome) was made, and the patient began treatment with prednisone, 1 mg/kg/day, and intravenous cyclophosphamide, 750 mg monthly for 6 months. No new neurologic symptoms developed after treatment was initiated, and strength in the hand and feet gradually improved over the subsequent year until she was able to walk independently without steppage.

Discussion: The presentation of a multifocal sensory and motor polyneuropathy (mononeuropathy multiplex) should immediately bring to mind the possibility of vasculitis, with a differential diagnosis of granulomatous disorders, lymphoma and other malignancies, and chronic infectious processes. Organ-specific vasculitis affecting peripheral nerve only can occur but is a diagnosis of exclusion. Any affected tissue can undergo biopsy, but if a nerve biopsy is to be performed, it is best to choose a nerve with, if possible, an abnormal but present sensory nerve action potential on testing. The yield of biopsy may be increased by performing a muscle biopsy using the same incision. Peripheral nerve vasculitis is a rapidly progressive, disabling, and treatable condition; therefore evaluation should proceed quickly.

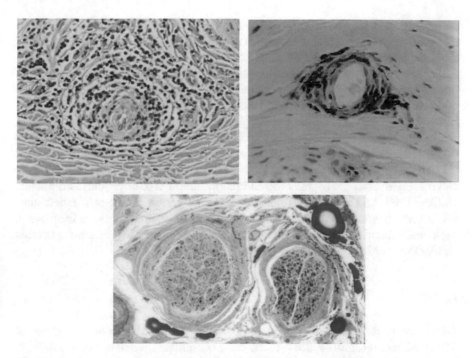

Fig. 5.3 Sural nerve biopsy demonstrating perivascular inflammatory infiltrates with transmural inflammation of epineurial vessels and axon loss that is variable in severity between nerve fascicles

Infiltrative disorders that can cause a mononeuropathy multiplex include lymphoma, carcinoma, and sarcoidosis. The etiologic diagnosis often rests upon biopsy of a nerve or another affected tissue. These conditions can also infiltrate nerve roots and the leptomeninges, in which case spinal fluid examination may provide either non-specific evidence of an inflammatory process, such as elevated protein, reduced CSF glucose, and a lymphocytic pleocytosis, or diagnostic findings, such as malignant cells on cytological examination or positive CSF Lyme serology.

Sarcoidosis may affect any portion of the neuroaxis. In the case of peripheral nerve, noncaseating granulomas infiltrate the nerve and cause perivascular inflammation [35]. Patients present with motor and sensory deficits, usually of acute onset, in named nerve distributions. Evidence of systemic disease is often present.

Treatment of mononeuropathy multiplex due to infiltrative disorders is generally the same as treatment of the etiologic process in other tissues.

Multifocal Motor Neuropathy and Lewis-Sumner Syndrome

Multifocal motor neuropathy (MMN) is an acquired multifocal immune-mediated neuropathy that exclusively affects motor nerves [36, 37]. The distal upper limbs are usually first affected, with ulnar, radial, and posterior interosseous nerves commonly affected. Most people with MMN have a slowly progressive course. CSF may show elevated protein, but it is usually normal, reflecting the fact that MMN typically affect intermediate or distal nerve segments more than the motor roots. Nerve conduction studies classically show conduction block in motor nerves, with normal sensory responses. In about 50% of cases, anti-GM1 ganglioside IgM antibodies are detected. Men are affected more often than women. The only medication shown to be effective in MMN is IVIg [16, 38].

Although MMN is classified as a distinct disorder, Lewis-Sumner syndrome (LSS) [39], or multifocal acquired demyelinating sensory and motor neuropathy (MADSAM [40]), is considered a variant of CIDP [36]. Unlike typical CIDP motor and sensory deficits are asymmetric and follow name nerve or plexus distributions. Unlike MMN, LSS affects both sensory and motor nerves. Nerve conduction studies in LSS show conduction velocity slowing or conduction block in focal nerve segments. Patients with LSS typically benefit from either IVIg or corticosteroids similar to typical CIDP.

HNPP

Although most hereditary neuropathies cause symmetric clinical deficits as discussed in the section on CMT, one notable exception is that of hereditary liability to pressure palsies (HNPP) [41]. HNPP is due to deletion of one copy of the PMP-22 gene. The mutation leads to reduced protein expression in nerve and subsequent thickened but faulty myelin (tomaculae). Affected patients develop isolated mononeuropathies, either with no identifiable cause or after brief periods of postural compression. Other presentations, including a reversible flail arm or even a length-dependent polyneuropathy pattern, can occur with HNPP. The diagnosis is suspected based upon a characteristic clinical history and electrodiagnostic examination and is confirmed by demonstration of a PMP22 deletion upon genetic testing. Treatment is currently focused upon avoidance of nerve compression.

Findings Isolated to One Limb

The discussion so far has focused on systemic neuromuscular disorders that usually affect more than one limb or body region. Some neuromuscular disorders, however, present with findings isolated to one limb. In such cases, the differential diagnosis is generally between a radiculopathy, plexopathy, and mononeuropathy (disease of an individual nerve). The examiner is therefore obliged to carefully examine the reflexes, distribution of sensory deficits, and individual muscle groups, all the while thinking carefully about which neuroanatomic structure is common to all of the abnormal findings. Radiculopathy, plexopathy, and mononeuropathy are usually due to extrinsic compression, trauma, or infiltration.

Radiculopathy

Patients affected with a radicular pattern of nerve injury can have injury to one or more nerve roots. Sensory symptoms often predominate, with pain or other positive phenomena originating in the neck or back and radiating down the affected limb. Numbness may be experienced in the corresponding dermatome. Due in part to the redundancy of root innervation of each muscle, weakness is less commonly experienced. If weakness occurs, a myotomal pattern might be appreciated. Careful evaluation of reflexes, looking not only for reflex loss but for reflex asymmetry, can provide helpful localizing information.

The most common causes of radiculopathy are extrinsic compression from herniated disk or foraminal osteophytes, most often at the C6-C7, C5-C6, L5-S1, and L4-L5 levels. Other causes of radiculopathy include infiltration from meningeal processes such as carcinomatous meningitis, lymphomatous meningitis, chronic meningeal infections, Lyme meningoradiculitis, meningeal sarcoidosis, and root avulsion due to trauma. Diabetes predisposes to acute thoracic and possibly lumbosacral radiculopathy as well and is discussed below. GBS and CIDP have a predilection for nerve roots and proximal segments of nerve and hence are most accurately referred to as polyradiculoneuropathies. While GBS and CIDP generally do not affect roots in isolation, there is an uncommon form of chronic inflammatory lumbosacral polyradiculopathy which, in many other respects including its response to immunotherapy, can be considered an anatomically restricted form of CIDP [32].

Plexopathy

Injuries to the plexus are far less common than those to nerve roots. The two primary plexuses affected are the brachial plexus and the lumbosacral plexus. Symptoms from plexopathy may include pain, weakness, and sensory loss in the distribution of the affected areas.

Neuralgic Amyotrophy (Parsonage-Turner Syndrome)

Neuralgic amyotrophy is a very distinct syndrome in that the presenting symptoms are quite similar in most patients and it is readily distinguishable from most other neurologic disorders. The characteristic presentation is severe acute pain in the shoulder region followed by weakness, atrophy, and sensory loss in the affected distributions. In most cases, this is a sensorimotor mononeuropathy multiplex affecting nerves of the shoulder girdle and upper limb. Commonly involved nerves include the long thoracic nerve, anterior interosseous nerve, and ulnar nerve, but any number of proximal and distal nerves of the region, including the phrenic nerve, can be involved [42]. Preceding events including trauma, exertion, or infection are common. The course is acute and monophasic, with recovery occurring over months to a year or more. Residual symptoms are not uncommon. Most often neuralgic amyotrophy is unilateral, but simultaneous or sequential involvement of both sides can occur. The pathogenic basis is not clearly established, but there is evidence of an immune-mediated process. Steroid therapy shortly after onset of symptoms can promptly alleviate pain and may accelerate recovery [43].

Hereditary Neuralgic Amyotrophy

Hereditary neurologic amyotrophy (HNA) is a rare group of familial disorders that present like neuralgic amyotrophy, except that multiple episodes occur during a lifetime. Some patients manifest non-neurologic findings including short stature, bifid uvula or cleft palate, syndactyly, and hypotelorism. Most cases of HNA are associated with mutations in the SEPT9 gene [44].

Diabetic Amyotrophy (Diabetic Radiculoplexus Neuropathy)

Patients with diabetes are susceptible to a distinct disorder of the lumbosacral roots and plexus known as *diabetic amyotrophy* or *diabetic radiculoplexus neuropathy* [45]. Much like neuralgic amyotrophy, which presents with acute, severe pain in the proximal upper limb, the common presentation of diabetic amyotrophy is acute, severe pain in the proximal lower limb, followed by weakness, numbness, and atrophy. Episodes may be associated with poorly controlled diabetes or rapid weight loss. The upper portions of the lumbosacral plexus and related lumbar roots are usually most severely affected. Because most people with this condition have a superimposed underlying diabetic neuropathy, differentiating chronic distal numbness and pain from a new plexus injury is sometimes challenging. Unilateral acute onset of pain in the thigh, groin, or low back followed by proximal weakness and atrophy of hip flexion or knee extension muscles (from upper lumbosacral plexus involvement) in a person with diabetes are clinical features suggesting diabetic amyotrophy. By contrast, diabetic polyneuropathy is bilateral and slowly progressive [45]. There is histologic evidence that it is vasculitic and some evidence that the natural history is improved by steroid therapy [45]. Like neuralgic amyotrophy, recovery in diabetic amyotrophy is slow, as it requires reinnervation, and is sometimes incomplete.

Plexopathy Associated with Mass

Any mass compressing the course of a plexus may produce plexopathy. Pain often occurs early, with weakness and sensory deficits evolving later. Neoplasm, hematoma, and abscess are important considerations. Assessment of the patient's risk factors (malignancy risk factors, anticoagulation medication, or predilection to infection) can provide important clues to the most likely etiology. For this reason imaging is a necessary component of the evaluation of plexopathy.

Radiation-Induced Plexopathy

Unlike plexus injured directly from a mass lesion, radiation-induced plexopathy typically causes gradually progressive weakness and sensory symptoms in the affected area, with less severe pain. Importantly, symptoms may develop months to years after radiation exposure. Despite these helpful historical distinctions between radiation-induced plexopathy and plexopathy from mass lesions, imaging remains imperative in these cases, not least because of the importance of excluding tumor recurrence. Radiation-induced plexopathy is likely due to tissue fibrosis and ischemia due to disruption of the microvascular architecture [46]. Several treatment algorithms designed to alleviate microvascular ischemia have been utilized, though none have a strong evidence base at the time of this writing.

Postoperative Plexopathies

Plexopathy is occasionally recognized in the postoperative period following open-heart surgery. Sternal retraction can lead to stretching or, in more severe cases, avulsion of the medial cord and lower trunk of the brachial plexus.

Diagnostic Testing for Brachial and Lumbosacral Plexopathy

Nerve conduction study and EMG can be very helpful for lesion localization. If a mass is suspected, CT or MRI of the plexus is essential. MRI with contrast can sometimes detect nerve signal change in those plexopathies that have an inflammatory mechanism. Clinical suspicion for malignant infiltration, infection, or inflammatory etiologies should trigger consideration of CSF analysis. Additional serologic work-up is guided by the clinical suspicion based upon a detailed history, taking into account the patient's unique circumstances.

Treatment of Cervical and Lumbosacral Plexopathy

Treatment is dictated by the underlying etiology. Immune-mediated processes may respond to corticosteroids, although this is unproven and generally only advised in the acute or subacute setting [47]. If a systemic condition or mass is uncovered (malignancy, abscess, or hematoma), treatment is focused upon the underlying disease process. Traumatic injuries may be treated by anastomosis of transected neural elements in severe cases, although this is generally ineffective for nerve root and lower trunk brachial plexus injuries. In many cases regardless of etiology, chronic management focuses on pain control and physical therapy to maintain or improve range of motion.

Mononeuropathies

The most common cause of mononeuropathies is compression: either repetitive, minor trauma (median entrapment at the wrist or carpal tunnel syndrome; ulnar entrapment at the elbow), single episodes of prolonged compression (radial neuropathy at the spiral groove; peroneal neuropathy at the fibular head), focal structural lesions, or HNPP. Infiltration of malignant or inflammatory cells can also cause mononeuropathies, particularly of the cranial nerves, as can vasculitis and other less common etiologies.

Compression, Entrapment, or Trauma

Median nerve compression at the wrist is the most common compressive neuropathy and results in carpal tunnel syndrome (CTS). Risk factors for CTS include repetitive hand use, obesity, pregnancy, endocrinopathy (hypothyroidism, diabetes), rheumatoid or osteoarthritis, and previous wrist fractures. Most patients experience pain in the wrist, paresthesias, and numbness of the hand and fingers (usually digits 1–3), as well as weakness of thumb abduction. Nerve conduction studies can characterize lesion localization and severity. Conservative treatment with wrist immobilization and nonsteroidal anti-inflammatory drugs (NSAIDs) is suggested for mild symptoms. In those with progressive weakness or refractory symptoms, surgical release of the transverse carpal ligament can be helpful and is ideally done before substantial motor axon loss develops [48].

The ulnar nerve is susceptible to injury in the antecubital fossa. Bone deformities (old fractures, arthritis), repetitive trauma, or soft tissue masses can cause or predispose to injury. Symptoms can be exacerbated by elbow flexion and may include pain at the elbow, paresthesias of the 4th and 5th digits, and weakness of hand intrinsic muscles, wrist flexion, and 4th and 5th digit flexion. Nerve conduction studies may reveal conduction velocity slowing or conduction block across the elbow. Mild cases may be managed medically with elbow protection. Surgical decompression or transposition may be considered if the injury is severe or refractory to conservative intervention [48].

Radial nerve injury most often occurs following proximal humerus fractures or sustained compression at the spiral groove (Saturday night palsy). Symptoms include weakness in wrist and finger extensors and sensory loss on the radial side of dorsal hand and thumb. Treatment with wrist splints for wrist support and to prevent contractures is important for mild injuries. Surgical exploration of injury site is indicated after severe trauma or after several months of failed medical management.

Femoral nerve injuries can occur due to compression from retroperitoneal or iliacus hematoma, pelvic or abdominal surgical positioning (lithotomy), inguinal ligament compression after prolonged hip flexion, or abduction with external rotation, childbirth, hip arthroplasty or dislocation, and trauma. Most patients only have weakness in knee extension, although if the lesion is above the inguinal ligament hip flexion weakness may also develop. Sensory loss affects the anteromedial thigh and medial calf (saphenous nerve). Nerve conduction studies may show a reduced femoral compound muscle action potential amplitude with an absent saphenous sensory response. If a retroperitoneal mass is suspected (abscess or hematoma), immediate CT imaging is of great importance. Treatment is guided by the underlying mechanism of injury and may include knee bracing, pain control, and surgical removal of any causative mass. Iliacus hematoma without trauma is a recognized complication of systemic anticoagulation and is often managed conservatively [49].

The lateral femoral cutaneous nerve is prone to compression as it emerges from underneath the inguinal ligament on the anterolateral thigh. Tight pants or belts and abdominal pannus are predisposing factors, but this commonly presents without an evident cause. Symptoms include neuropathic pain, paresthesias, and sensory loss over the lateral thigh and are virtually pathognomonic. Weakness does not occur. Management includes weight loss and avoidance of compressive clothing. Neuropathic pain can be treated topically if the affected area is not too large. The condition is referred to as *meralgia paresthetica*.

Common peroneal, superficial peroneal, and deep peroneal neuropathies are usually due to external compression (prolonged bed rest, surgical positioning, or prolonged leg crossing or squatting), structural pathology at the fibular head (cysts or tumors), or fibular fracture or knee dislocation. *Rapid weight loss in the absence of a history of compression is a recognized cause of acute peroneal neuropathy as well.* Symptoms include weakness of ankle eversion (superficial peroneal branch) and dorsiflexion (deep peroneal branch). Sensory loss may affect the anterolateral lower leg and foot dorsum (superficial peroneal nerve) or 1st and 2nd digit webspace (deep peroneal nerve). Nerve conduction studies may reveal conduction block or conduction velocity slowing across the fibular head (mild, early) or reduced peroneal amplitude (late, with axon loss). The superficial peroneal sensory nerve response may be absent or reduced if the superficial peroneal branch is involved. Treatment depends upon the mechanism of injury but often includes lateral and posterior knee protection.

Diabetes: A Special Case

Diabetes is the most common cause of distal, symmetric, sensory-predominant polyneuropathy, which sometimes presents before diabetes is evident or when the patient has only impaired glucose tolerance or impaired fasting glucose [50]. *Diabetes can also cause mononeuropathies. The following mononeuropathies are common in people with diabetes*:

- Cranial mononeuropathies: CN III, VI, and VII are most common. Diabetic CN III palsies are often associated with a normal papillary response, unlike compressive third nerve palsy from an expanding aneurysm.
- Thoracic radiculopathy.
- Limb mononeuropathy:

- Median at the wrist
- Ulnar at the elbow
- Peroneal at the fibular head

The term "diabetic neuropathy" is generally meant to refer to the distal symmetric polyneuropathy associated with diabetes. Focal or generalized weakness in a person with diabetes is, until proven otherwise, either a diabetic mononeuropathy, diabetic radiculoplexopathy, or something else unrelated to diabetes. It is important to avoid the trap of diagnosing all neuromuscular problems in people with diabetes as "diabetic neuropathy," because many focal or generalized peripheral nerve disorders, even in a diabetic, are managed differently than diabetic distal symmetric polyneuropathy.

Neuropathies Associated with Monoclonal Gammopathies

Monoclonal gammopathy (paraproteinemia) is the overproduction of a single monoclonal immunoglobulin (M protein) from a clone of B lymphocytes or plasma cells. Approximately 10% of patients with idiopathic peripheral neuropathy have monoclonal proteins. The neuropathies associated with monoclonal gammopathy can be extremely variable in presentation [51, 52].

Monoclonal Gammopathy of Undetermined Significance (MGUS)

Although IgG is the most common Ig class causing a serum paraprotein, when associated with neuropathy, IgM is more frequent (60%), followed by IgG (30%) and IgA (10%) [52]. Neuropathies with IgG or IgA monoclonal protein can be demyelinating (like CIDP) or axonal (like length-dependent sensorimotor axonal polyneuropathy). IgM-associated neuropathy is more often demyelinating, frequently with a DADS phenotype [20].

Multiple Myeloma

Multiple myeloma-associated neuropathy is usually distal, axonal, and sensory or sensorimotor [53]. Nerve conduction studies and nerve biopsy reveal evidence of axonal degeneration. The paraprotein is usually IgG or IgA, with γ or μ heavy chain or κ light chain. Systemic features include bone pain, weight loss, fatigue, anemia, and hypercalcemia. Lytic bone lesions may be seen on a skeletal survey. The diagnosis is made by bone marrow biopsy showing greater than 10% plasma cells. Treatment consists of treatment of myeloma.

Amyloidosis

Amyloidosis may be acquired or hereditary [54]. *Acquired amyloidosis* can be primary or associated with other lymphoproliferative conditions such as multiple myeloma, Waldenstrom's macroglobulinemia, or lymphoma. Early disruption of autonomic function and small fiber modalities (painful dysesthesias with loss of pin and temperature sensation) is common. A paraprotein is present in 90% and can be IgA, IgM, or IgG, usually with a λ light chain. Nerve biopsy reveals loss of small fibers and amyloid deposits with Congo red stain. Soft tissue biopsy (e.g., fat, rectal, kidney) may also reveal amyloid deposits. *Hereditary amyloidosis* is associated with mutations in transthyretin (TTR), apolipoprotein A-1, or gelsolin genes. TTR mutations are the most common. Like the acquired forms, small fiber and autonomic symptoms are common, and soft tissue biopsy may show amyloid deposits. Unlike acquired forms, the clinical course is slower, and M proteins are not present. The diagnosis of hereditary amyloidosis is made by genetic testing. Amyloidosis must be considered in any idiopathic acquired sensorimotor polyneuropathy with autonomic symptoms or unexplained pain.

POEMS Syndrome

POEMS syndrome is a paraneoplastic syndrome driven by neoplastic plasma cells [55]. The acronym refers to the symptoms and signs that predominate: polyneuropathy, organomegaly, endocrinopathy, M protein (IgG or IgA lambda light chain), and skin changes. In over 75% of patients, osteosclerotic myeloma is present. POEMS syndrome can also develop in angiofollicular lymph node hyperplasia (Castleman's syndrome). In up to 50%, polyneuropathy is the presenting feature. Sensory and motor symptoms begin distally and extend proximally in an acute to subacute (weeks to months) time course. NCS may be indistinguishable from CIDP. CSF protein levels and serum VEGF levels are often markedly elevated [56]. It is important to consider POEMS in the appropriate clinical context because it is associated with a rapidly progressive disabling polyneuropathy, and treatment of the underlying malignancy can lead to clinical stabilization or improvement.

Waldenstrom's Macroglobulinemia

Waldenstrom's macroglobulinemia is a lymphoplasmacytoid malignancy with a prominent clonal production of IgM. Systemic features include fatigue, weight loss, hemorrhages, anemia, and lymphadenopathy. The associated neuropathy is usually a sensory-predominant large fiber polyneuropathy affecting the hands and feet [57]. Gait imbalance and sensory ataxia may be severe. The paraprotein is usually an IgM κ, and one third of patients also have anti-MAG antibodies. Nerve conduction studies show evidence of demyelination, often with profound distal latency prolongation. Nerve biopsy reveals demyelination and myelin membrane IgM deposits. Bone marrow shows the malignant lymphoplasmacytoid cells. Treatment is directed toward the primary malignancy.

Cryoglobulinemia

Cryoglobulins are proteins against polyclonal immunoglobulins that precipitate at reduced temperatures. Cryoglobulinemia can occur as a consequence of a primary lymphoproliferative disorder or secondary to chronic inflammatory processes, most notably chronic hepatitis C infection. The systemic features of cryoglobulinemia include organomegaly, renal failure, purpura, and arthralgia. The associated neuropathy is usually painful with either a length-dependent or mononeuropathy multiplex pattern [58]. Nerve conduction studies and EMG reveal evidence of axon loss. Nerve biopsy may show axon loss, necrotizing vasculitis, or inflammatory infiltration. Treatment with corticosteroids, cyclophosphamide, or PLEX may be helpful for the neuropathy. When it is secondary to chronic hepatitis C infection, eradication of the underlying infection is essential as well.

Summary

When approaching a new patient with suspected neuropathy, it is often tempting to initiate an exhaustive and unfocused diagnostic odyssey. If the diagnostician has a fundamental understanding of the modalities affected, pattern of involvement, and temporal evolution, the investigative process can instead be focused on the most likely etiologies. Specific causes of polyneuropathy, some of which have been discussed above, can be explored with precision, and treatment approaches can be developed with a focus on the underlying etiology.

References

1. Barohn RJ. Approach to peripheral neuropathy and neuronopathy. Semin Neurol. 1998; 18(1):7–18.
2. Barohn RJ, Amato AA. Pattern-recognition approach to neuropathy and neuronopathy. Neurol Clin. 2013;31(2):343–61.
3. Hughes R. Peripheral nerve diseases: the bare essentials. Pract Neurol. 2008;8(6):396–405.
4. Krause SJ, Backonja MM. Development of a neuropathic pain questionnaire; Clin J Pain. 2003;19:306–14.
5. Devigili G, Tugnoli V, Penza P, Camozzi F, Lombardi R, Melli G, et al. The diagnostic criteria for small fibre neuropathy: from symptoms to neuropathology. Brain. 2008;131:1912–25.
6. Tesfaye S, Boulton AJM, Dyck PJ, Freeman R, Horowitz M, Kempler P, et al. Diabetic neuropathies: update on definitions, diagnostic criteria, estimation of severity, and treatments. Diabetes Care. 2010;33:2285–93.
7. Hughes RAC, Umapathi T, Gray IA, Gregson NA, Noori M. A controlled investigation of the cause of chronic idiopathic axonal polyneuropathy. Brain. 2004;127:1723–30.
8. Smith AG, Singleton JR. Obesity and hyperlipidemia are risk factors for early diabetic polyneuropathy. J Diabet Complicat. 2013;27:436–42.
9. Terkelsen AJ, Karlsson P, Lauria G, Freeman R, Finnerup NB, Jensen TS. The diagnostic challenge of small fiber neuropathy: presentations, evaluations, and causes. Lancet Neurol. 2017;16:934–44.

10. Finnerup NB, Attal N, Haroutounian S, McNichol E, Baron R, et al. Pharmacotherapy for neuropathic pain in adults: a systematic review and meta-analysis. Lancet Neurol. 2015;14:162–73.
11. Vallat JM, Mathis S, Funalot B. The various Charcot-Marie-Tooth diseases. Curr Opin Neurol. 2013;26(5):473–80.
12. Gutmann L, Shy M. Update on Charcot-Marie-Tooth disease. Curr Opin Neurol. 2015;28(5):462–7.
13. McGrath MC. Charcot-Marie-Tooth 1A: a narrative review with clinical and anatomical perspectives. Clin Anat. 2016;29(5):547–54.
14. Reilly MM, Murphy SM, Laura M. Charcot-Marie-Tooth disease. J Peripher Nerv Syst. 2011;16:1–14.
15. Van den Bergh PY, Hadden RD, Bouche P, et al.; European Federation Neurological Societies; Peripheral Nerve Society. European Federation of Neurological Societies/Peripheral Nerve Society guideline on management of chronic inflammatory demyelinating polyradiculoneuropathy: report of a joint task force of the European Federation of Neurological Societies and the Peripheral Nerve Society – first revision. Eur J Neurol. 2010;17(3):356–63.
16. Joint Task Force of the EFNS and the PNS. European Federation of Neurological Societies/Peripheral Nerve Society guideline on management of multifocal motor neuropathy. Report of a joint task force of the European Federation of Neurological Societies and the Peripheral Nerve Society—first revision. J Peripher Nerv Syst. 2010;15(4):295–301.
17. Mahdi-Rogers M, Brassington R, Gunn AA, van Doorn PA, Hughes RA. Immunomodulatory treatment other than corticosteroids, immunoglobulin and plasma exchange for chronic inflammatory demyelinating polyradiculoneuropathy. Cochrane Database Syst Rev. 2017;5:CD003280.
18. Hughes RA, Donofrio P, Bril V, Dalakas MC, Deng C, et al. Intravenous immune globulin (10% caprylate-chromatography purified) for the treatment of chronic inflammatory demyelinationg polyradiculoneuropathy (ICE study): a randomized placebo-controlled trial. Lancet Neurol. 2008;7:136–44.
19. Kuwabara S, Mori M, Misawa S, Suzuki M, Nishiyama K, et al. Intravenous immunoglobulin for maintenance treatment of chronic inflammatory demyelinating polyneuropathy: a multicenter, open-label, 52-week phase III trial. J Neurol Neurosurg Psychiatry. 2017;88:832–8.
20. Katz JS, Saperstein DS, Gronseth G, Amato AA, Barohn RJ. Distal acquired demyelinating symmetric neuropathy. Neurology. 2000;54(3):615–20.
21. Vital A, Vital C, Julien J, Baquey A, Steck AJ. Polyneuropathy associated with IgM monoclonal gammopathy. Immunological and pathological study in 31 patients. Acta Neuropathol. 1989;79:160–7.
22. Willison HJ, Jacobs BC, van Doorn PA. Guillain-Barré syndrome. Lancet. 2016;388(10045):717–27.
23. Fokke C, van den Berg B, Drenthen J, et al. Diagnosis of Guillain-Barré syndrome and validation of Brighton criteria. Brain. 2014;137:33–43.
24. Verboon C, van Doorn PA, Jacobs BC. Treatment dilemmas in Guillain-Barré syndrome. J Neurol Neurosurg Psychiatry. 2016. [Epub ahead of print].
25. González-Suárez I, Sanz-Gallego I, Rodríguez de Rivera FJ, Arpa J. Guillain-Barré syndrome: natural history and prognostic factors: a retrospective review of 106 cases. BMC Neurol. 2013;13:95.
26. van Doorn PA. Diagnosis, Treatment, and Prognosis of Gullain-Barre Syndrome. Presse Med 2013;42:193–201.
27. Hiraga A, Mori M, Ogawara K, et al. Recovery patterns and long term prognosis for axonal Guillain-Barré syndrome. J Neurol Neurosurg Psychiatry. 2005;76(5):719–22.
28. Shahrizaila N, Kokuun N, Sawai S, Umapathi T, Chan YC, et al. Antibodies to single glycolipids and glycolipid complexes in Guillain-Barre syndrome sybtypes. Neurology 2014;83:118–24.
29. Susuki K, Yuki N, Schafer DP, Hirata K, Zhang G, Funakoshi K, Rasband MN. Dysfunction of nodes of Ranvier: a mechanism for anti-ganglioside antibody-mediated neuropathies. J Peripher Nerv Syst. 2014;19:115–20.
30. Mori M, Kuwabara S, Fukutake T, Yuki N, Hattori T. Clinical features and prognosis of Miller Fisher syndrome. Neurology. 2001;56(8):1104–6.
31. Gwathmey KG. Sensory neuronopathies. Muscle Nerve. 2016;53(1):8–19.

32. Caporale CM, Staedler C, Gobbi C, Bassetti CL, Uncini A. Chronic inflammatory lumbosacral polyradiculopathy: a regional variant of CIDP. Muscle Nerve. 2011;44:833–7.
33. Collins MP, Arnold WD, Kissel JT. The neuropathies of vasculitis. Neurol Clin. 2013;31(2): 557–95.
34. Hehir MK 2nd, Logigian EL. Infectious neuropathies. Continuum (Minneap Minn). 2014;20(5 Peripheral Nervous System Disorders):1274–92.
35. Fritz D, van de Beek D, Brouwer MC. Clinical features, treatment and outcome in neurosarcoidosis: systematic review and meta-analysis. BMC Neurol. 2016;16(1):220.
36. Allen JA, Parry GJ. Acquired Immunologic Neuropathies. Semin Neurol. 2015;35(4):398–406.
37. Nobile-Orazio E. Multifocal motor neuropathy. J Neuroimmunol. 2001;115(1–2):4–18.
38. Umapathi T, Hughes RA, Nobile-Orazio E, Léger JM. Immunosuppressant and immunomodulatory treatments for multifocal motor neuropathy. Cochrane Database Syst Rev. 2015;(3):CD003217.
39. Lewis RA, Sumner AJ, Brown MJ, Asbury AK. Multifocal demyelinating neuropathy with persistent conduction block. Neurology. 1982;32:958–64.
40. Saperstein DS, Amato AA, Wolfe GI, Katz JS, Nations SP, et al. Multifocal acquired demyelinating sensory and motor neuropathy: the Lewis-Sumner syndrome. Muscle Nerve. 1999;22:560–6.
41. van Paassen BW, van der Kooi AJ, van Spaendonck-Zwarts KY, Verhamme C, Baas F, de Visser M. PMP22 related neuropathies: Charcot-Marie-Tooth disease type 1A and Hereditary Neuropathy with liability to Pressure Palsies. Orphanet J Rare Dis. 2014;9:38.
42. Sumner AJ. Idiopathic brachial neuritis. Neurosurgery. 2009;65(4 Suppl):A150–2.
43. Van Alfen N, van Engelen BG, Hughes RA. Treatment for idiopathic and hereditary neuralgic amyotrophy (brachial neuritis). Cochrane Database Syst Rev. 2009;(3):CD006976.
44. van Alfen N. Clinical and pathophysiological concepts of neuralgic amyotrophy. Nat Rev Neurol. 2011;7(6):315–22.
45. Dyck PJ, Windebank AJ. Diabetic and nondiabetic lumbosacral radiculoplexus neuropathies: new insights into pathophysiology and treatment. Muscle Nerve. 2002;25(4):477–91.
46. Pradat PF, Delanian S. Late radiation injury to peripheral nerves. Handb Clin Neurol. 2013;115:743–58.
47. van Alfen N, van Engelen BG, Hughes RA. Treatment for idiopathic and hereditary neuralgic amyotrophy (brachial neuritis). Cochrane Database Syst Rev 2009;(3):CD006976.
48. Hobson-Webb LD, Juel VC. Common entrapment neuropathies. Continuum. 2017;23:487–511.
49. Tosun A, Inal E, Keles I, Tulmac M, Tosun O, Aydin G, Orkun S. Conservative treatment of femoral neuropathy following retroperitoneal hemorrhage: a case report and review of the literature. Blood Coagul Fibrinolysis. 2014;25:769–72.
50. Smith AG, Rose K, Singleton JR. Idopathic neuropathy patients are at high risk for metabolic syndrome. J Neurol Sci. 2008;273:25–8.
51. Joint Task Force of the EFNS and the PNS. European Federation of Neurological Societies/ Peripheral Nerve Society Guideline on management of paraproteinemic demyelinating neuropathies. Report of a joint task force of the European Federation of Neurological Societies and the Peripheral Nerve Society – first revision. J Peripher Nerv Syst. 2010;15(3):185–95.
52. Nobile-Orazio E. Neuropathy and monoclonal gammopathy. Handb Clin Neurol. 2013;115:443–59.
53. Kelly JJ, Kyle RA, Miles JM, et al. The spectrum of peripheral neuropathy in myeloma. Neurology. 1981;31:24–31.
54. Shin SC, Robinson-Papp J. Amyloid neuropathies. Mt Sinai J Med. 2012;79(6):733–48.
55. Dispenzieri A. POEMS syndrome: 2014 update on diagnosis, risk-stratification, and management. Am J Hematol. 2014;89(2):214–23.
56. D'Souza A, Hayman SR, Buadi F, et al. The utility of plasma vascular endothelial growth factor levels in the diagnosis and follow-up of patients with POEMS syndrome. Blood. 2011;118(17):4663–5.
57. Levine T, Pestronk A, Florence J, et al. Peripheral neuropathies in Waldenström's macroglobulinemia. J Neurol Neurosurg Psychiatry. 2006;77:224–8.
58. Santoro L, Manganelli F, Briani C, Giannini F, Benedetti L, Vitelli E, et al. HCV Peripheral Nerve Study Group. Prevalence and characteristics of peripheral neuropathy in hepatitis C virus population. J Neurol Neurosurg Psychiatry. 2006;77:626–629.

Chapter 6
The Diagnostic Approach to the Hypotonic and Weak Infant

Peter I. Karachunski

Abbreviations

CMD   Congenital muscular dystrophy
SMA   Spinal muscular atrophy

Key Points
- Hypotonia is a common and nonspecific presentation of dysfunction of the nervous system in children of early age.
- Hypotonic infant is non-localizing presentation which makes differentiation between central and peripheral processes difficult.
- Diagnosis of a specific neuromuscular disorder is based on a pattern recognition of muscle weakness, constellation of ancillary testing followed by genetic testing for targeted gene or panel of relevant genes.
- Early diagnosis of spinal muscular atrophy is of great importance as there is available treatment which showed best results in presymptomatic infants.
- Specific diagnosis of congenital myopathic disorders is critical for prognostication, guiding treatments, genetic counseling, and readiness for participation in clinical studies.
- Multidisciplinary approach in management of neuromuscular patients is critical to address multiorgan and multisystem involvement frequently seen in very young patients.

Introduction

The hypotonic infant is a common neurological problem encountered in the setting of neonatal intensive care and outpatient pediatric neurology practice. In infancy, unlike in older patients, hypotonia alone is non-localizing but can reflect pathology

P.I. Karachunski, MD (✉)
University of Minnesota, Department of Neurology, Minneapolis, MN, USA
e-mail: karac001@umn.edu

© Springer International Publishing AG, part of Springer Nature 2018
D. Walk (ed.), *Clinical Handbook of Neuromuscular Medicine*,
https://doi.org/10.1007/978-3-319-67116-1_6

at any location in the central or peripheral nervous system. In addition, all newborn infants with serious systemic illness such as congenital heart disease, sepsis, and others can present with hypotonia. Thus, identifying hypotonia in infancy is only the first step in the diagnostic process [1].

The Diagnostic Evaluation of the Hypotonic Infant

Physical and Neurological Examination

The prenatal history may provide valuable diagnostic clues. A history of reduced fetal movements and polyhydramnios often indicates muscle weakness in utero. The perinatal history is important as well, with an emphasis on respiratory function and capacity for latching during breastfeeding.

A general physical examination should be performed to evaluate for presence of deformities such as pectus excavatum, plagiocephaly (flattening of the occipital region of the skull as a result of lying in one position for extended periods of time), arthrogryposis (congenital contractures), characteristic craniofacial changes such as dolichocephaly and high-arched palate, and fish-like shape of the mouth, which is frequently open at rest. Attention should be paid to other dysmorphic features.

It is important to observe how the infant is breathing. Usually, an infant with weakness does not show overt signs of respiratory distress such as increased work of breathing, retraction, or nasal flaring. Instead, infants with respiratory muscle weakness will appear calm with tachypnea, shallow breathing, and abdominal breathing, in which abdominal muscles play an accessory role in the respiratory effort.

The neurological examination of an infant begins with simply observing the infant's behavior at rest. Special attention is paid to the state of alertness, resting posture, spontaneous motor activity, and the presence of adventitious movements. In particular, it is important first to determine the state of alertness in an infant during examination. A sleeping infant or an infant with a reduced level of consciousness is likely to demonstrate hypotonia and hyporeflexia as a reflection of their level of consciousness rather than neuromuscular disease.

The cranial nerve examination in the infant is essentially an evaluation of brainstem reflexes, as outlined in Table 6.1. Note in particular that assessment of suck and swallow is an important part of the neuromuscular examination of the infant. A speech pathologist with expertise in evaluation of infants can assist in this as well.

Motor Examination

The motor examination of the newborn is performed in supine, prone, and upright (vertical) positions.

Table 6.1 Cranial nerve examination in the newborn

Cranial nerve	Test
II, III	Pupillary reaction to light
III, IV, VI (EOMs)	Oculocephalic maneuver
V	Corneal reflex Masseter reflex
VII	Spontaneous facial grimacing Lip reflex to lip tapping Glabella reflex to glabellar tapping
VII, VIII	Acoustic blink reflex to clapping
IX, X	Gag reflex
XI	Head positioning and movements
XII	Tongue protrusion, movements, and bulk
IX, X, XII	Suck reflex

Supine

In the supine position, a healthy infant maintains their legs in a semi-flexed position at the knees with slight abduction at the hips, while a hypotonic infant's legs are fully abducted at the hips such that the lateral aspect of the thigh touches the surface of an exam table. A healthy infant's arms are flexed at the elbows in the supine position, while they are extended in the hypotonic infant.

Prone

Examination of the infant in the prone position is performed by grasping the baby with both hands at the thorax and suspending the infant horizontally in the prone position, known as "ventral suspension." A healthy infant will attempt to lift the head and draw the legs to the abdomen against gravity. A hypotonic and weak baby cannot produce this effort and appears with the head, upper, and lower extremities hanging, forming a "C" shape (Fig. 6.1). If an infant is placed on the surface in prone position, spontaneous crawling can be initiated and can be further enhanced by providing light pressure to its feet (Bauer's response).

Upright

The *traction response* is evaluated by grasping the supine infant's hands and pulling the infant toward the sitting position. In a healthy term infant, the head will follow the movement of the body by rising and maintaining posture. By contrast, in a hypotonic infant, the head will lag behind the body while the torso is pulled forward. In addition, an examiner will notice a degree of resistance during flexing of the upper extremities in normal infants; this is reduced in the hypotonic infant. This response is also reduced in premature infants and is absent in infants of less than 33 weeks

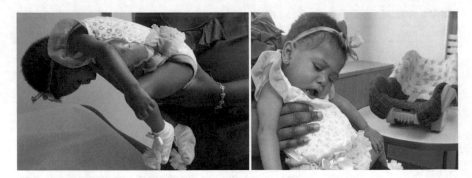

Fig. 6.1 Hypotonic child with inability to elevate the head in the prone or upright position

Table 6.2 Motor examination of the newborn infant

Position	Maneuver	Normal	Abnormal
Supine	Lying	Flexed leg posture	Frog-leg posture
	Traction	Attempt to lift the head	Head lag
Prone	Lying	Flexed posture with head turned to one side	Inability to lift or turn the head
	Lying	Spontaneous crawling and with tactile reinforcement (Bauer's response)	Lack of spontaneous crawling or Bauer's response
	Suspended	Antigravity posture with head control and flexed extremities	Lack of postural control; the head and extremities hang
Upright	Suspended	Placing response: Foot is lifted with flexion in the knee and hip followed by extension after dorsum of the foot placed under the edge of the table	Absence of placing response
	Suspended	Touching the feet on the surface stimulates stepping movements	No stepping movements

gestational age. Another bedside test is called *vertical suspension*. This test is performed by lifting the infant at the axillae without grasping the chest. Muscle strength and tone of the shoulders should be sufficient to prevent the baby from slipping through examiner's hands. The head should be upright and legs drawn up in a flexed position. The hypotonic infant's extremities will remain flaccid with the head dropped. The examiner immediately appreciates the necessity of holding the baby tight, grasping for the thorax.

Central Hypotonia

Central hypotonia is due to dysfunction of the upper motor neuron, which occurs in disorders of the brain and, less commonly, the spine. Hypotonia due to brain disorders is frequently accompanied by other signs of cerebral dysfunction such as altered mental status, seizures, or movement disorder. The relative preservation of muscle strength, which can be evidenced by postural reflexes, normal or increased deep tendon reflexes, clenched fists, or cortical thumb sign, strongly suggests a central rather than peripheral cause of hypotonia.

Common causes of central hypotonia include the following:

- Hypoxic-ischemic encephalopathy
- Chromosomal disorders, such as Prader-Willi, Angelman, Down, Noonan, fragile X, and Turner's syndromes
- Genetic disorders, such as familial dysautonomia, oculocerebrorenal syndrome, peroxisomal disorders, mitochondrial diseases, and inborn errors of metabolism
- Brain malformations
- Intrauterine infections

Central hypotonia is more common than peripheral hypotonia [2].

Peripheral Hypotonia

Peripheral hypotonia refers to hypotonia due to disorders of the motor unit including the low motor neuron, peripheral nerves, neuromuscular junction, or muscle. *Peripheral hypotonia is always accompanied by weakness.* In general, disorders of the motor unit are less likely to be associated with congenital organ malformations. Exceptions include disorders with both peripheral and central nervous system involvement such as can be seen in congenital muscular dystrophies or disorders of peroxisomal biogenesis. Other abnormalities may include the presence of congenital contractures or arthrogryposis. Facies can be dysmorphic with fish-like mouth appearance, small jaw, micrognathia, and dolichocephaly. Prenatal history is often remarkable for reduced fetal movements, polyhydramnios, and some level of respiratory or nutritional support needed at birth.

On examination, infants with peripheral causes of hypotonia lie with their legs splayed apart and with reduced or absent spontaneous movements. The degree of hypotonia is consistent with the infant's ability to move spontaneously and in response to stimulation. Deep tendon reflexes are diminished or absent; by contrast, robust reflexes in the context of hypotonia are suggestive of a central cause. While a nonspecific finding, muscle bulk may be reduced. Fasciculations can be limited to superficial muscles such as the tongue and, when present, are highly suggestive of a disorder of motor neurons. Postural reflexes such as tonic neck, Moro, and Galant reflexes are depressed or absent as well.

Diagnostic Evaluation of Suspected Disorders of the Motor Unit

Ancillary tests are used in the diagnosis of peripheral hypotonia to confirm a clinical suspicion of a disorder of the motor unit and further characterize the underlying pathological process and etiology. Common confirmatory tests in this context are listed below:

- Molecular diagnostics
- Electrodiagnostic study
- Histopathological analysis
- Biochemical markers
- Imaging of muscles and peripheral nerves (MRI, ultrasound)
- Pharmacological testing

Molecular Diagnostics

In the last decade, DNA-based testing has become the first line in many clinical scenarios including evaluation of the hypotonic infant. This is attractive because of its affordability, specificity, and noninvasive nature. Most conditions in which peripheral hypotonia is a prominent feature can be diagnosed by carrying out genetic testing alone. The approach may include one or multiple single-gene analyses, a panel using next-generation sequencing analysis, or whole exome sequencing. The most common conditions tested include spinal muscular atrophy, myotonic dystrophy, and some forms of muscular dystrophies.

Electrodiagnostic Study

Electromyography (EMG) and nerve conduction studies (NCS) remain an important asset for additional characterization of the process and localization. A distinct benefit of EMG and NCS is that it can be performed at the bedside, and results are available immediately. Nonetheless, performing electrodiagnostic study in a very young child can be a very difficult task and is best when performed by an experienced physician. Both EMG and NCS can provide invaluable diagnostic information and are especially helpful in differentiating neurogenic from myopathic processes. While normal EMG and NCS do not rule out involvement of the motor unit, normal results are very uncommon in a severely affected infant with a neuromuscular disorder.

There are several features of EMG and NCS that are unique to very young pediatric patients. Because of incomplete myelination, conduction velocities are very slow and can mask demyelinating neuropathy. Nerve conduction velocities increase in a predictable fashion as a child ages and reach adult values between 3 and 5 years of age. Motor units tend to be smaller and are fewer per muscle, which makes compound muscle action potential amplitudes smaller. On needle examination, motor unit action potentials are of lower amplitudes and of smaller duration, which can be mistaken for myopathic features. Because infants cannot voluntarily contract to command, interpretation of recruitment pattern can be difficult. Spontaneous activity such as fibrillation potentials and fasciculations may be relatively subtle and of lower amplitude as well. Specialized testing for abnormalities of neuromuscular transmission can be obtained including repetitive nerve stimulation and single-fiber EMG. The latter is done using a stimulation technique in this population because of lack of cooperation.

Histopathological Evaluation

Muscle biopsy can be performed at any age but can be technically challenging in very young infants. In the past, muscle biopsy played a critical role in the diagnosis of infants with hypotonia. Muscle biopsy is no longer needed to diagnose several conditions that can be confirmed with genetic testing. Muscle biopsy can, however, provide important information in cases where genetic testing is negative or inconclusive. Choice of a biopsy site is important but may be not as critical as in older individuals where the process can be patchy and sampling error is more common. Nerve biopsy is rarely performed in very young children [3].

Biochemical Testing

Serum creatine kinase (CK) should be performed in all hypotonic infants. When increased, a myopathic process with involvement of skeletal and, less commonly, cardiac muscle is likely. While mild elevation in CK can be seen in neuropathic processes as well, this is seen less commonly in very young children than in adults. Newborn infants can have increased CK level from birth asphyxia or other systemic illness associated with acidosis. Therefore, repeated measurements of serum CK may be required to confirm the significance of such an elevation. A normal CK does not rule out a myopathic disorder but reduces the likelihood of a disorder associated with muscle fiber loss, such as muscular dystrophy. Other markers include lactic acid, which may be increased in mitochondrial disorders. Its elevation is not specific and can be caused by other systemic disorders associated with acidosis. Therefore, it is not very diagnostic as an isolated finding. Testing for carnitine and acyl-carnitine profiles, amino acids, and urine organic acids may be helpful for cases where a metabolic cause of muscle hypotonia is suspected.

Imaging

Because of associated finding of brain malformation or T2 signal abnormalities in some conditions, brain MRI should be obtained in these patients. This is especially important when congenital muscular dystrophy is suspected. Imaging is diagnostic in very rare cases of anterior horn disease such as pontocerebellar hypoplasia.

Direct imaging of the muscle can be done with ultrasound or MRI. Muscle ultrasound is a very simple bedside technique that can be done in conjunction with electrodiagnostic studies and can be used to demonstrate both abnormal echogenicity, as is seen when the muscle is replaced by fat and connective tissue, and spontaneous muscle activity such as fasciculations.

Pharmacological Testing

The Tensilon test can be used to assess the response to edrophonium chloride (Tensilon®) when a disorder of neuromuscular transmission is suspected. Edrophonium chloride is a rapidly acting anticholinesterase compound that temporarily reverses weakness in disorders of neuromuscular transmission such as myasthenia gravis. This test is rarely used in neonates. Reversal of muscle weakness is very difficult to verify in neonates; furthermore, patients with congenital myasthenic syndromes such as AChE deficiency and abnormalities in ColQ, Dok-7, MuSK, agrin, LRP4, plectin, and laminin β2 can show no improvement, or even worsening, in response to AChE inhibitors. Therefore, it should be used with caution and in appropriately selected cases only.

Selected Neuromuscular Disorders that Can Present as a Hypotonic Infant

Disorders of Anterior Horn Cells

Spinal Muscular Atrophy

Spinal muscular atrophy (SMA) is the most common disorder of anterior horn cells in children. SMA is an autosomal recessive disorder with a homozygous deletion of exons 7 and 8 of the SMN1 (survival motor neuron) gene on chromosome 5q13 in about 95% cases. The remaining 5% are compound heterozygous for deletion of exons 7 and 8 or a point mutation of the other SMN1 allele [4]. In the most severe case such as Werdnig-Hoffman disease, or SMA type 1, symptoms begin in the first 6 months of life. In some cases in which motor neuron degeneration begins in utero, decreased fetal movements can be perceived. Such infants present with severe hypotonia at birth and respiratory failure requiring mechanical ventilation. Less severely affected infants develop progressive hypotonia and weakness with involvement of skeletal muscle, proximal greater than distal. Hypotonia and weakness can be striking and are rapidly progressive when onset is in the first 6 months of life. Bulbar and respiratory dysfunction result in lack of weight gain due to dysphagia, loss of motor milestones, and ventilatory failure. Cardinal findings are tongue fasciculations and atrophy, which in combination with areflexia are seen in all infants with SMA type 1 are essentially pathognomonic for this condition. Infants with apparent respiratory insufficiency demonstrate paradoxical breathing frequently described as "abdominal." This occurs when there is relative sparing of the diaphragm in comparison to thoracic accessory respiratory muscles. Despite the severity of their motor symptoms, these infants appear very alert, which can be a very striking feature of SMA type 1.

While variable from child to child, the course of SMA is very predictable and depends on the age of onset of symptoms. Infants with presentation at birth will likely die within first 6 months of life without significant support. Some infants may achieve some milestones such as rolling or even sitting but will lose them shortly thereafter. If untreated, almost all infants with SMA type 1 do not survive for more than 2 years. The prognosis of SMA is changing, thanks to nusinersen, which is explained below.

When there is high level of clinical suspicion, the diagnosis of SMA should be confirmed by genetic testing [4]. Currently, the testing is commercially available and has a rapid turnaround time. This precludes invasive tests such as NCS/EMG and muscle biopsy. When immediate information is necessary however, a needle EMG can be obtained and always demonstrates evidence of a neuropathic process, including fibrillation potentials, fasciculation potentials, and reduced recruitment with large motor unit action potentials. Muscle biopsy is almost never done to confirm a diagnosis of SMA currently. If obtained, muscle biopsy findings are striking and demonstrate grouped atrophy. Routine histological stains show groups of small fibers of either type and groups of hypertrophic fibers that are almost always type 1.

Genetic testing in SMA demonstrates zero copies of the SMN1 gene and at least one copy of the SMN2 gene. The SMN2 gene differs from SMN1 by substitution of one codon in exon 7, which acts as a silencer of exon splicing. The resulting SMN2 product is a nonfunctional truncated version of the SMN1 gene product. However, small amounts of a functional SMN protein are made from an alternative splicing of SMN2, and this modifies the SMA phenotype. Thus, more copies of SMN2 are associated with a milder phenotype. Typically, patients with SMA type 1 have two or three copies of the SMN2 gene. Patients with later-onset SMA (types 2 and 3) have three, four, or even five copies of the SMN2 gene.

It is imperative to make a diagnosis of SMA early because of the recent FDA approval of Nusinersen, a treatment for SMA. This medication is based on antisense oligonucleotide technology and suppresses the exon silencer of SMN2, resulting in increased production of SMN protein. Individuals with higher SMN2 copy number have a better response to nusinersen. Data from clinical trials demonstrated significant efficacy, which led to FDA approval for patients with at least two copies of SMN2 [5]. The benefit of this medication is greatest in least affected or presymptomatic infants. Nusinersen is administered intrathecally and requires repeat injection every 4 months. Other genetic treatments for SMA may soon be available as well [6].

The advent of nusinersen notwithstanding, supportive therapies are necessary for infants with respiratory failure. This includes noninvasive or invasive ventilation, insufflation-exsufflation (cough assist) treatment, and airway clearance with a vibrating vest. Dysphagia and insufficient nutritional intake require gastrostomy placement.

Other Causes of SMA

When an infant with suspected SMA has negative genetic testing for an SMN1 gene deletion, the differential diagnosis includes a number of rare disorders, which can be confirmed by molecular analysis utilizing next-generation sequencing or whole exome sequencing. In some cases there are additional diagnostic clues suggesting an alternative diagnosis. For example, in infants with distal-predominant weakness and respiratory failure, spinal muscular atrophy with respiratory distress (SMARD1) should be suspected. This disorder is due to a mutation in the immunoglobulin μ-binding protein 2 (IGHMBP2) [7]. Other features of SMARD1 include sparing of intercostal respiratory muscles, greater involvement of upper extremities and distal muscles, early respiratory failure, and mild contractures. The course is usually rapidly progressive. SMARD2 is an X-linked disorder due to a mutation in the ribosomal biogenesis protein LAS1L [8]. Another rare disorder associated with anterior horn cell degeneration is pontocerebellar hypoplasia (PCH) [9]. Imaging of the brain in this condition demonstrates marked hypoplasia of the pons and cerebellum. Only types 1A and 1B are associated with SMA. These infants can present at birth or later in infancy and have a progressive course. Metabolic causes of SMA should be considered as well. These include mitochondrial disorders such as cytochrome-c oxidase deficiency, which is classically described as a cardioencephalomyopathy syndrome but can have variable presentations, including SMA. A diagnostic clue is the presence of multisystem involvement including encephalopathy with seizures, skeletal myopathy, and cardiomyopathy. On examination, ptosis and ophthalmoplegia are characteristic. One rare treatable metabolic disorder associated with anterior horn cell involvement is Brown-Vialetto-van Laere syndrome (BVVL), which is an autosomal recessive riboflavin transporter disorder caused by mutations in SLC52A2 and SLC52A3 genes [10]. This disorder can present in a variable fashion with more severe cases presenting with rapid onset of bulbar weakness and respiratory failure in infancy. Hearing loss is a significant clue to the diagnosis of BVVL. Other features include sensory neuropathy, optic nerve atrophy, and central hypoventilation and apnea. Treatment with high doses of riboflavin is very effective in slowing or halting progression.

Disorders of Peripheral Nerves

Peripheral neuropathies are rarely encountered as a cause of peripheral hypotonia in infants. They can be divided into axonal and hypomyelinating forms, based upon the primary pathological process. Significant axon loss is seen in familial dysautonomia syndrome (Riley-Day syndrome), which is due to a mutation in the gene for inhibitor of κ-light polypeptide gene enhancer in B cells, kinase complex-associated protein (IKAP) [11]. This can present with congenital onset of hypotonia with lack of tears, areflexia, absence of lingual fungiform papillae, and axonal flare after intradermal histamine. Pain insensitivity, gastrointestinal dysfunction, hyperhidrosis and autonomic crises occur as well. Riley-Day syndrome has an increased prevalence in Ashkenazi Jews. Congenital hypomyelinating polyneuropathy is an infantile or early-onset form of Charcot-Marie-Tooth disease. Recognized forms include an autosomal recessive or dominant mutation in myelin protein 0 (MPZ), allelic with CMT1B, CMT2I and 2 J, and CMT4E, which is due to autosomal recessive or dominant mutations in the early growth response 2 gene (EGR2; KROX20). Infants with congenital hypomyelinating neuropathy present with severe hypotonia, areflexia, and weakness which includes the facial muscles. Nerve conduction velocities are very slow and do not improve with time.

Myopathic Disorders

Congenital Myotonic Dystrophy

Congenital myotonic dystrophy (DM) is an uncommon autosomal dominant disorder due to a large CTG triplet repeat expansion in the DMPK gene. The size of the repeat expansion directly correlates with the age of onset of myotonic dystrophy and is typically >700 CTG triplet repeats in congenital DM [12]. Such infants are usually born to an affected mother due to an anticipation phenomenon, which does not occur when inherited from the father. During the pregnancy a history of polyhydramnios, decreased fetal movements, breech presentation, and premature labor is common. The mother of a baby with congenital DM generally has a relatively mild form of myotonic dystrophy and is frequently diagnosed at the time of the infant's birth. The main manifestation of congenital DM is severe hypotonia and weakness resulting in minimal motor activity, respiratory failure, and bulbar dysfunction with inability to suck, swallow, and control secretions. Facial dysmorphism characterized by dolichocephaly, fish-like mouth, and high-arched palate is a common finding as well. Neurological examination shows facial diplegia, opened mouth with inverted V shape, and bilateral ptosis with normal extraocular movements and pupillary response to light. Reduced gag reflex, hypophonia or aphonia, and shallow breathing, which frequently requires respiratory support, are also typical findings in neonatal onset of congenital DM. Deep tendon reflexes are almost always absent. Multisystem dysfunction can accompany muscle weakness and includes gastroparesis and cardiac involvement. Neonatal mortality can be significant without respiratory and nutritional support. When a diagnosis of congenital myotonic dystrophy is suspected, a brief examination of the mother can be very helpful. While not always striking, facial features may be revealing and consistent with facial weakness, ptosis, and bitemporal muscle wasting (temporal dimpling) (Fig. 6.2). The presence of clinical myotonia and myotonic discharges on electromyography in the mother is essentially diagnostic of this disorder when suspected in the infant. Electromyography of the child, by contrast, can be helpful but not diagnostic. It is characterized by findings of an irritable myopathy but without myotonic discharges. The diagnosis is confirmed by molecular analysis, which will show a large CTG repeat expansion.

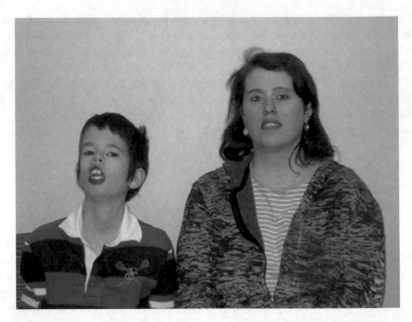

Fig. 6.2 Mother and child with myotonic dystrophy, demonstrating the phenomenon of anticipation

Management of congenital DM consists of respiratory support with invasive or noninvasive approaches, nutritional support with tube feeding, and evaluation and treatment of cardiac complications. Most infants who survive the neonatal period will show improvement and stabilization with little or no need for ventilatory support. Most will acquire the ability to ambulate independently but with persistent distal-predominant weakness. Complex cognitive dysfunction of varying severity is present in all children with congenital onset of this disorder.

Congenital Muscular Dystrophy

Congenital muscular dystrophy (CMD) is a heterogeneous group of muscle disorders with onset of hypotonia and weakness in the neonatal period [13]. Most causes of CMD are inherited in an autosomal recessive fashion, with some presenting as autosomal dominant conditions typically due to a de novo mutation. Typically infants with CMD present with diffuse weakness and hypotonia resulting in respiratory compromise and bulbar dysfunction. Many have congenital contractures (arthrogryposis) or hyperlaxity. Most infants with CMD present with a static course initially followed by gradual deterioration over many years, with the exception of SEPN1- and RYR1-related muscular dystrophy. The majority of infants with CMD are not able to attain independent ambulation.

In the current classification system, CMD is grouped in several categories based on molecular features and genetic abnormalities. Subtypes of CMD include, laminin alpha 2-related dystrophies (merosin-deficient CMD), α-dystroglycan-related

CMDs (muscle-eye-brain disease), collagen VI-related dystrophies, SEPN1-related CMD, RYR1-related CMD, LMNA-related CMD, and CMD which is not genetically classified. Diagnostically these disorders are distinguished by associated findings, such as brain abnormalities often evident on MRI in disorders of glycosylation and merosin-deficient CMD. Elevated CK is a common finding in CMDs with the exceptions of SEPN1, RYR1, and collagen VI-related disorders, where it can be normal or mildly abnormal. EMG is nonspecific and is characterized by features of an irritable myopathy. Muscle pathology shows dystrophic features including fiber size variation, necrosis and degeneration of muscle fibers, and significant fibrosis. Muscle MRI or ultrasound may provide supportive information in the early phase of the diagnostic evaluation. The following is a discussion of the most common forms of CMDs [13].

LAMA2-CMD (Laminin Alpha 2 or Merosin-Deficient CMD, MDC1A)

Neonatal onset of this disorder is characterized by diffuse hypotonia, weakness, contractures, and elevated CK level. Contractures can affect hands and feet, consistent with arthrogryposis. The complete deficiency of the protein will preclude independent ambulation, while in children with partial deficiency, independent ambulation can be achieved. Brain MRI shows very striking changes with abnormal high signal in the white matter seen on T2 and FLAIR sequences (Fig. 6.3). This finding can be pathognomonic if correlated to the appropriate clinical phenotype and CK level. Additional findings may include occipital cortical dysgenesis associated with heterotopia and cerebellar hypoplasia. As many as 30% of patients will develop epilepsy. Most patients have normal cognitive development.

α-Dystroglycan-Related CMD

This is a heterogeneous group of disorders caused by mutations in as many as 18 genes involved in the glycosylation pathway. Because of the normal abundance of α-dystroglycan in the brain and muscle, involvement of these organs is primarily responsible for the phenotype. The spectrum of severity of brain malformation is broad and most severe among patients presenting in the neonatal period. Classic phenotypes present as muscle-eye-brain disease with severe malformation of the brain, including cobblestone lissencephaly seen in Walker-Warburg syndrome, muscle-eye-brain disease in Fukuyama CMD due to mutations in fukutin (FKTN) gene, focal pachygyria, occipital cortical dysplasia with a smooth-appearing cortex and an underlying heterotopic band of neurons, midbrain hypoplasia, pontocerebellar hypoplasia, and cerebellar hypoplasia with and without cerebellar cysts. Muscle hypotonia and weakness with diffuse involvement are also seen in patients with congenital onset. A milder syndrome can occur as well, presenting as limb-girdle muscular dystrophy or with a phenotype similar to Duchenne and Becker muscular dystrophy. Cardiac monitoring should be considered for all patients with dystroglycanopathies, especially those with muscular dystrophies due to fukitin-related protein (FKRP) and FKTN gene mutations.

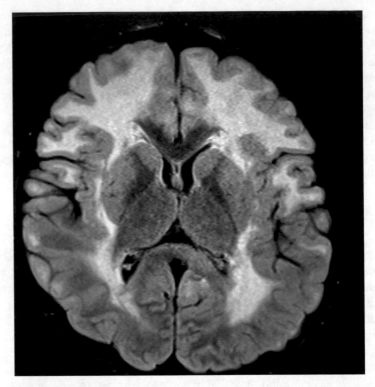

Fig. 6.3 FLAIR sequence of brain MRI demonstrating diffuse T2 hyperintensity in the white matter with abnormal gray matter thickening of the posterior-inferior occipital lobes

Collagen VI (COL6)-Related Muscular Dystrophies

COL VI-related muscular dystrophies can present with a spectrum of severity of phenotypes from severe early-onset congenital muscular dystrophy (Ullrich CMD) to mild distal-predominant Bethlem myopathy. Congenital onset is characterized by severe generalized hypotonia and weakness with prominent hyperlaxity of wrists, joints of the fingers, and ankles. Many infants present with hip dislocation. Contractures at the elbows and knees may be evident at birth and progress over the course of the disease. Later in the course of the disease, intermediate joints of phalanges develop contractures as well. Kyphoscoliosis is an early complication, which is seen in all patients with congenital onset. Motor milestones are significantly delayed, but many infants develop new motor skills. Some patients can achieve independent ambulation, which is lost later in life. Significant restrictive lung disease progresses gradually, making patients dependent on nocturnal noninvasive ventilatory support due to markedly disproportionate involvement of the diaphragm. More severely affected patients may even require continuous ventilatory support.

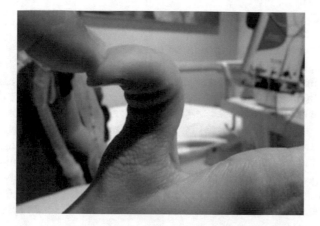

Fig. 6.4 Hyperlaxity in an adult with collagen VI-related muscular dystrophy

In addition to contractures and hyperlaxity in joints (Fig. 6.4), the skin can be affected with keratosis pilaris and abnormal scarring with keloid and parchment paper-like formation. The diagnosis is based on clinical findings, normal or mildly elevated CK, and characteristic imaging findings by ultrasound, with a central shadow pattern in the muscle.

SEPN1-Related Myopathy

SEPN1-related myopathy is an autosomal recessive congenital muscle disorder due to a mutation in the SEPN1 gene encoding for selenoprotein N. This disorder rarely presents with severe neonatal hypotonia, feeding difficulty, and respiratory failure. The most striking feature in an affected infant is a significant head lag out of proportion to muscle tone and strength of other muscle groups. Despite some delay in motor development, such infants will continue to show an improvement in muscle strength and will acquire milestones and the ability to ambulate independently. Hyperlaxity in the digits and wrists is noticeable in infancy, but development of contractures is not a prominent feature, with the exception of a rigid spine, which becomes evident later in life. Respiratory failure requiring noninvasive respiratory support may be significant and can develop while the patient remains ambulatory. Facial involvement is minimal and restriction in extraocular motions is not commonly seen. Ancillary testing demonstrates normal or mildly elevated CK, a myopathic EMG pattern, and a multiple minicore pattern on muscle biopsy which is evident on oxidative enzyme stains and, in particular, NADH stain. This pattern consists of multiple pale areas in the muscle fibers depleted of mitochondria and internal architecture. It is not pathognomonic and can be seen in other myopathic disorders such as RYR1-related myopathy. The specific diagnosis is made via genetic testing.

Recessive RYR1-Related Myopathy

While RYR1-related myopathy can be inherited in both recessive and dominant fashion, congenital onset occurs in the former. In congenital onset RYR1-related myopathy, muscle hypotonia and weakness are evident at birth and can be associated with difficulty in feeding and respiratory insufficiency. Mechanical ventilation usually is not required, however. Mild facial and ocular involvement can be seen but is not always distinct and easy to diagnose in infants. Severe scoliosis can develop, typically after 5 years of age. The diagnosis is based on clinical findings, normal or mildly elevated CK, and genetic testing. Muscle biopsy can be helpful in diagnosis but is not specific as it can present with different patterns including central core, multiple minicore, fiber-type disproportion, extreme fiber atrophy, prominent central nucleation, and significant fibrosis with relatively minimal degenerative and regenerative fibers.

LMNA-Related CMD

CMD due to a recessive mutation in the lamin A/C (LMNA) gene is an uncommon form of muscular dystrophy and is one of many clinical phenotypes caused by abnormalities in this gene, including the classic phenotype of Emery-Dreifuss muscular dystrophy. In congenital onset there is overt generalized hypotonia and weakness with superimposed severe weakness of the axial and neck muscles resulting in characteristic "head drop syndrome," which can be pathognomonic in the appropriate clinical setting (Fig. 6.1). These infants can have difficulties with swallowing that may require tube feeding. Respiratory insufficiency often requires noninvasive nocturnal respiratory support but not invasive mechanical ventilation. One of the major concerns is an arrhythmogenic cardiomyopathy, which may require treatment with an automatic implantable defibrillator device. CK is mildly to moderately increased. Cognition is normal. The diagnosis is based on clinical findings and genetic testing. Muscle biopsy pattern can demonstrate a variety of findings ranging from fiber type 1 atrophy to overtly dystrophic features characterized by degenerating and necrotic fibers with some features of inflammation and fibrosis. Immunochemistry is not helpful as lamin A/C staining is always present in the congenital form (Table 6.3).

Congenital Myopathies

The *congenital myopathies* are a heterogeneous group of disorders with onset of muscle hypotonia and weakness at birth and early infancy. *They are distinguished by the presence of at least one typical pathological pattern in the muscle biopsy and the absence of features of degenerative muscles disease, such as degenerating and necrotic fibers, inflammation, and significant fibrosis.* Congenital myopathies range in severity from profound weakness resulting in akinesia and arthrogryposis incompatible with survival to a mild presentation with delay in gross motor milestones only.

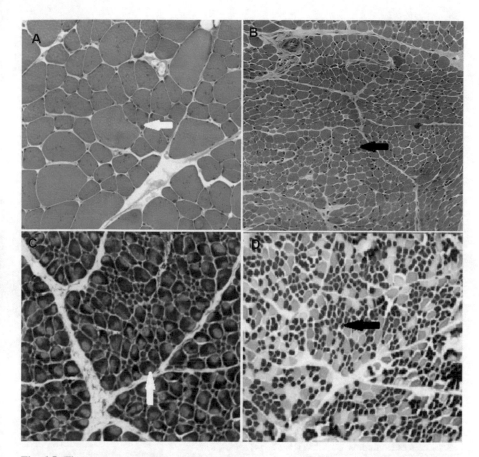

Fig. 6.5 The most common histopathological patterns in muscle biopsy from patients with congenital myopathies. **A**. Gomori-Trichrome stain of the muscle with characteristic pattern of darkly stained intracellular rods (white arrow) found in patient with nemaline myopathy due to AR mutations in the nebulin gene. **B**. H&E stain shows numerous atrophic fibers in contrast to normal size fibers. Many atrophic fibers have central nuclei (black arrow) such as seen in centronuclear myopathy due to mutation in the MTM1 gene. **C**. NADH stain with atrophic fibers and larger fibers with an area of reduced staining – cores (white arrow) – as seen in congenital myopathy due to mutation in the nebulin gene. **D**. ATPase staining used for fiber typing shows all darkest stained fibers very small (black arrow). This pattern is consistent with fiber type disproportion which in this case is due to a mutation in the RYR1 gene

The course is typically very slowly progressive or static. In the past congenital myopathies were classified according to classic histological patterns (Fig. 6.5) [14]; in recent years, however, it has become clear that each histologic pattern of congenital myopathy may reflect one of several mutations [15]. Various pathophysiologic mechanisms have been implicated, including disorders of sarcolemmal and intracellular membrane remodeling and excitation-contraction coupling, mitochondrial

Table 6.3 Congenital muscular dystrophies – pattern recognition

CMD type	Pattern of muscle weakness	CK increase	MRI brain abnormality	Cardiomyopathy	Joint involvement
LAMA2	Diffuse	++	T2 increase, cortical dysgenesis	None	Early contractures, arthrogryposis
α-Dystroglycan disorders	Diffuse, proximal	++	Malformations	Yes (FKRP, FKTN)	Arthrogryposis
Collagen VI disorders	Core > respiratory > proximal	+/−	None	None	Hyperlaxity of distal joints, proximal contractures
SEPN1	Core, head drop	+/−	None	None	Hyperlaxity, rigid spine later
RYR1	Core, bulbar, respiratory	+/−	None	Yes	Severe scoliosis later
LMNA	Core, head drop, bulbar, respiratory	++	None	Yes	Contractures > weakness

Table 6.4 Histopathological patterns seen in congenital myopathies

Histopathological classification	Mutated gene
Nemaline rods	ACTA1, NEB, TPM2, TPM3, TNNT1, CFL-2, KBTBD13, KLHL40, KLHL41
Central cores	RYR1, SEPN1, ACTA1, TTN, CFL-2, DNM2, MYH7, MYH2
Central nuclear	MTM1, DNM2, BIN1, RYR1, CCDC78, SPEG, TTN
Multicores or minicores	RYR1, SEPN1, NEB,TTN
Fiber-type disproportion	ACTA1, TPM2, TPM3, SEPN1, MYH7, RYR1, HACD1

distribution and function, disturbances of myofibrillar force generation, and autophagy. Lack of specificity in clinicopathological correlation of congenital myopathies has led to use of next-generation sequencing as first-line testing in many clinical scenarios of infants who present with hypotonia and weakness (Table 6.4) [16].

Disorders of Neuromuscular Transmission

Disorders of neuromuscular transmission are the most uncommon cause of hypotonia in infancy. They are divided into acquired and genetic causes. *Acquired causes* include neonatal myasthenia gravis and botulism. The former occurs due to passive transfer of antibodies via the placenta into an infant, causing transient symptoms of fatigable weakness involving bulbar, ocular, and respiratory muscles. Rarely, the diagnosis of autoimmune myasthenia gravis is not known in the mother before onset of the symptoms in an infant. This typically resolves within several weeks. Treatment includes pyridostigmine and, in severe cases, IVIg or PLEX. Botulism is a presynaptic disorder that has onset several weeks to months after birth and presents with progressive weakness, constipation, hypotension, hypohidrosis, and mydriasis. Treatment includes supportive therapy and use of botulism immune globulin.

Congenital myasthenic syndromes (CMS) are a heterogeneous group of genetic disorders caused by mutations in more than 30 genes [17]. The forms of CMS are classified by mechanism of action including disorders of presynaptic, synaptic, and postsynaptic functions, disorders of protein glycosylation in the neuromuscular junction (NMJ), and abnormalities in development and maintenance of the NMJ. The most common cause of CMS is a primary AChR deficiency, accounting for more than 30% of cases. The other common causes of CMS include primary AChR kinetic abnormality, rapsyn deficiency, end-plate AChR deficiency, and DOK7 deficiency. Together these disorders account for about 90% of all CMS. CMS are unified by a common presentation [17]. Most present at birth with fluctuating fatigable weakness affecting ocular, bulbar, respiratory, and skeletal muscles. A variable degree of support is required, including noninvasive and invasive ventilatory support and tube feeding. The diagnosis is based on the constellation of clinical findings and is confirmed by repetitive nerve stimulation and single-fiber EMG, which demonstrate an abnormal decrement and increased jitter characteristic of disorders of neuromuscular transmission. It is important to further characterize the precise cause of CMS with genetic testing. Knowledge of the underlying genetic cause may provide an understanding of the pathophysiology and guide choice of appropriate medications for treatment of CMS.

Conclusion

The clinical presentation of congenital hypotonia is a challenging diagnostic problem and requires integration of clinical findings, when indicated, with a combination of electrodiagnostic techniques, serological testing, muscle and brain imaging, histopathological analysis of muscle, and genetic testing. Targeted genetic testing is becoming increasingly prevalent as a first-line diagnostic test once the most likely diagnoses are established based upon clinical criteria. Identifying the specific etiologic diagnosis in an infant with a congenital neuromuscular disorder is important not only for prognostication and genetic counseling but for guiding treatment.

References

1. Volpe JJ. Neonatal hypotonia in neuromuscular disorders of infancy, childhood, and adolescence a clinical approach. 2015. p. 85–94.
2. Fenichel GM. Clinical pediatric neurology: a signs and symptoms approach. 6rd ed. The hypotonic Infant. 2009. p. 153–176.

3. Dubowitz V, Sewry CA. Muscle biopsy. A practical approach. 3rd ed. 2007.
4. Bharucha-Goebel D, Kaufmann P. Treatment Advances in Spinal Muscular Atrophy. Curr Neurol Neurosci Rep 2017;17:91.
5. Mercuri E, et al. Diagnosis and management of spinal muscular atrophy: part 1: recommendations for diagnosis, rehabilitation, orthopedic and nutritional care. Neuromuscul Disord. 2017;(17):31284–1.
6. Mendell JR, Al-Zaidy A, Shell R, Arnold WD, Rodino-Klapac LR. Single-dose gene replacement therapy for spinal muscular atrophy. N Engl J Med. 2017;377:1713–22.
7. Litvinenko I, Kirov AV, Georgieva R, Todorov T, Malinova Z, Mitev V, Todorova A. One novel and one recurrent mutation in IGHMBP2 gene, causing severe spinal muscular atrophy respiratory distress 1 with onset soon after birth. J Child Neurol. 2014;29:799–802.
8. Butterfield RJ, Stevenson TJ, Xing L, Newcomb TM, Nelson B, et al. Congenital lethal motor neuron disease with a novel defect in ribosome biogenesis. Neurology. 2014;15:1322–30.
9. Rudnik-Schoneborn S, Barth PG, Zerres K. Pontocerebellar hypoplasia. Am J Med Genet Semin. 2014;166C:173–83.
10. Karachunski P, Dalton J, Molero-Ramirez H, Grames M. A case of childhood onset of treatable sensory neuronopathy caused by mutations in riboflavin transporter RFVT2 presenting as pure sensory ataxia with excellent response to riboflavin – a five year follow up. Neuromuscul Disord. 2017;27:S206.
11. Rubin BY, Anderson SL. The molecular basis of familial dysautonomia: overview, new discoveries, and implications for directed therapies. NeuroMolecular Med. 2008;10:148–56.
12. Yum K, Wang ET, Kalsotra A. Myotonic dystrophy: disease repeat range, penetrance, age of onset, and relationship between repeat size and phenotypes. Curr Opin Genet Dev. 2017;44:30–7.
13. Fu X-N, Xiong H. Genetic and clinical advances in congenital muscular dystrophy. Chin Med J. 2017;130:2624–31.
14. Sewry CA, Wallgren-Pettersson C. Myopathology in congenital myopathies. Neuropathol Appl Neurobiol. 2017;43:5–23.
15. Ravenscroft G, Laing NG, Bonnemann CG. Pathophysiological concepts in the congenital myopathies: blurring the boundaries, sharpening the focus. Brain. 2015;138:246–68.
16. Ravenscroft G, Davis MR, Lamont P, Forrest A, Laing NG. New era in genetics of early-onset muscle disease: breakthroughs and challenges. Semin Cell Dev Biol. 2017;64:160–70.
17. Engel AG, Shen XM, Selcen D, Sine SM. Congenital myasthenic syndromes: pathogenesis, diagnosis, and treatment. Lancet Neurol. 2015;14:420–34.

Chapter 7
Rehabilitation Therapists' Role in Management of Neuromuscular Disease

Robin Samuel

Abbreviations

AAC	Augmentative and alternative communication
AD	Assistive device
ADLs	Activities of daily living
AFO	Ankle-foot orthosis
ALS	Amyotrophic lateral sclerosis
ALS-CBS	ALS Cognitive Behavioral Screen
ALSFRS-R	ALS Functional Rating Scale-Revised
ATP	Assistive technology practitioner
CMT	Charcot-Marie-Tooth
EADLs	Electronic aids to daily living
FVC	Forced vital capacity
IADLs	Instrumental activities of daily living
IBM	Inclusion body myositis
LE	Lower extremity
MCP	Metacarpophalangeal joint
MMD	Myotonic muscular dystrophy
NMD	Neuromuscular disease
OT	Occupational therapist
PLS	Primary lateral sclerosis
PT	Physical therapist
ROM	Range of motion
SLP	Speech-language pathologist
UE	Upper extremity

R. Samuel (✉)
University of Minnesota Health, Fairview Rehabilitation Services,
Minneapolis, MN, USA
e-mail: Rsamuel1@fairview.org

© Springer International Publishing AG, part of Springer Nature 2018
D. Walk (ed.), *Clinical Handbook of Neuromuscular Medicine*,
https://doi.org/10.1007/978-3-319-67116-1_7

133

Key Points
- Rehabilitation therapists help people cope with functional impairments associated with neuromuscular disease.
- Impairments vary with each type of neuromuscular disease.
- Each person requires an individualized approach.
- Rate of progression of disease is varied.
- Occupational and physical therapists and speech-language pathologists are key members of a multidisciplinary team.
- Mobility, assistive devices, and lower extremity orthoses need to be addressed.
- Home accessibility is a key component of helping people with neuromuscular disease plan for progression.
- ADL/IADL, assistive technology, adaptive equipment, and orthoses are important components that need to be addressed with neuromuscular disease.
- Functional vision can be affected with some neuromuscular diseases.
- Fatigue and respiratory and cardiac function are affected in many forms of neuromuscular disease.
- Exercise, spasticity management, and contracture prevention require an individualized approach based on current research associated with disease processes.
- Dysarthria, dysphagia, and augmentative and alternative communication need to be addressed for functional communication and safe and adequate oral nutrition.
- Cognition and behavior need to be assessed as part of comprehensive care of people with neuromuscular disease.
- Caregivers benefit from training to understand how to best provide care and support their loved ones with neuromuscular disease.

Introduction

Neuromuscular disease (NMD) leads to many changes in daily living skills, mobility, speech, and swallowing. These arise from impairments specific to the type of NMD. These impairments affect function and are best addressed by rehabilitation therapists who are familiar with NMD. Treatment requires an individualized approach as each disease process is different, resulting in different impairments. Within a given type of disease, rate of progression varies as well. People benefit from early and ongoing assessment and treatment by rehabilitation therapists. Occupational therapists (OTs), physical therapists (PTs), orthotists, hand therapists, and speech-language pathologists (SLPs) help people live with the functional impairments that are associated with NMD. Therapists also teach caregivers as their loved ones become more dependent on others in managing daily activities and mobility. Therapists' roles are to improve function with an eye toward quality of life, safety, independence, and symptom management.

The World Health Organization's International Classification of Functioning, Disability and Health distinguishes between impairments (problems in body

Table 7.1 Common impairments in NMD and their functional consequences

Impairment	Activity limitation	Disability
Sensory loss	Standing without tactile input	Cannot attend large gatherings
Proximal weakness	Walking >100 ft	Cannot visit shopping malls
Diplopia	Reading	Cannot participate in school
Hand weakness	Grasping, using utensils	Cannot prepare food
Diaphragm weakness	Breathing supine	Cannot sleep in bed
Reduced shoulder range of motion	Reaching behind trunk	Cannot dress or bathe independently
Spastic dysarthria	Cannot speak rapidly or clearly	Cannot use a telephone effectively
Impaired swallowing	Sialorrhea, choking	Avoids social events centered around meals

function or structure), activity limitations (problems in execution of activities), and disability (an outcome of the interaction between health conditions and contextual factors (environmental and personal participation)) [1]. Table 7.1 lists examples of impairments in NMD and their consequences.

In addition to these largely concrete physical limitations, the additional effort required to complete simple tasks such as self-care and walking, musculoskeletal pain, non-restorative sleep, and the psychological impact of impairments from NMD result in an added burden of fatigue, which itself has concrete functional consequences.

Key Members of a Multidisciplinary Team

Physical, occupational, and speech therapists are critical members of a multidisciplinary neuromuscular team. Therapy evaluation and intervention may occur as part of a multidisciplinary clinic visit, in a therapy clinic, during an inpatient rehabilitation stay, or at home. The definitions and scope of practice of therapy specialties are outlined below. Table 7.2 provides general examples of key areas assessed and the impact on function.

Occupational Therapy (OT) Role

The American Occupational Therapy Association defines OT as "the therapeutic use of everyday life activities (occupations) with individuals or groups for the purpose of enhancing or enabling participation in roles, habits, and routines in home, school, workplace, community, and other settings." [2]. *Note that, in this context, "occupation" refers not to employment but to everyday life activities that enable*

Table 7.2 General roles of the three therapy specialties commonly utilized in NMD

Specialty	Assessments	Function
Physical therapy	Trunk and lower body function Muscle tone Posture Balance Gait	Mobility
Occupational therapy	Upper body function Dexterity Endurance Cognition Vision	Daily living activities
Speech-language pathology	Speech Voice Augmentative communication Swallowing	Communication Oral nutrition

one's life roles. These "occupations" are subdivided into activities of daily living (ADLs), instrumental activities of daily living (IADLs), and other categories [2]. Many OTs also use the term electronic aids to daily living (EADLs) to refer to the ever-expanding use of technology to control electronic devices in the environment for daily living.

- ADLs: basic self-care such as brushing teeth, eating, dressing, and taking a shower.
- IADLs: tasks that support daily life at home and in the community. Specific IADLs may include caring for others, meal preparation, driving, shopping, and managing finances and health.
- EADLs: use of technology for daily living.
- Other occupations: rest and sleep, education, work, play, leisure, and social participation.

OTs assess the whole person by addressing impairments in the areas of vision, cognition, behavior, physical abilities, and coping skills. OTs look at meaningful roles and "occupations" a person has in their life and how impairments are impacting these occupations, in order to help a person compensate or adapt.

Physical Therapy (PT) Role

The American Physical Therapy Association describes PTs as "health care professionals who help individuals maintain, restore, and improve movement, activity, and functioning, thereby enabling optimal performance and enhancing health, well-being, and quality of life." [3] PTs generally assess and manage the following domains in NMD:

- Joint range of motion
- Strength and endurance

- Spasticity
- Musculoskeletal pain
- Turning, transferring, standing, and walking
- Balance

In addition to making assessments and recommendations in these domains, PTs advise on the use of durable medical equipment, including gait aids, transfer and lift devices, wheelchairs, and power mobility. With NMD, PTs' focus of intervention is often to improve safety and efficiency of mobility.

Speech-Language Pathologist (SLP) Role

The American Speech-Language-Hearing Association defines a SLP as "the professional who engages in professional practice in the areas of communication and swallowing across the life span." [4] SLPs assist in the following:

- Evaluating swallowing at the bedside or via a videofluoroscopic swallowing study
- Recommending diet modifications and safe swallowing strategies
- Evaluating and treating speech and voice dysfunction
- Recommendations and training for augmentative communication devices
- Evaluating language and cognitive disorders that impact communication

Orthotist Role

The American Board for Certification in Orthotics, Prosthetics and Pedorthics defines an orthotist as "an allied health professional specifically educated and trained to make and fit orthoses and prostheses and manage comprehensive orthotic and/or prosthetic patient care." [5] In the context of NMD, orthotists work principally with ankle-foot orthoses, upper extremity splints, and neck supports.

Hand Therapist Role

The American Society of Hand Therapists defines a hand therapist as "an occupational or physical therapist who, through advanced continuing education, clinical experience and integration of knowledge in anatomy, physiology and kinesiology, has become proficient in treatment of pathological upper extremity conditions resulting from trauma, disease, congenital or acquired deformity." [6] In the context of NMD, hand therapists fit custom upper extremity splints, recommend exercises for range of motion in hands, and recommend adaptations for upper extremity or hand function. They are generally called upon as subspecialists to supplement OT or orthotist's skills.

Functional Assessment and Intervention in OT, PT, and SLP

Assessments

Therapists are trained in a wide range of validated assessments of impairment and disability. These assessments are extraordinarily valuable as they provide objective information that informs clinical decision-making. In the context of the time limitations of medical practice, therapists' assessments also greatly extend providers' ability to understand their patients' needs and provide independent information not biased by the physician-patient relationship. Table 7.3 lists many validated assessment tools commonly used in NMD clinics.

In addition, there is a growing number of validated patient-reported functional assessments for longitudinal assessment in NMD, some typically administered by a trained evaluator and some validated for patient completion. A list of these is included in the Appendix.

Interventions

Mobility, Assistive Devices, and Lower Extremity Orthoses

Mobility refers to walking, operating a wheelchair, or transferring from one surface or position to another. Mobility is impacted by whole-body strength, range of motion, sensation, muscle tone, balance, and respiratory and cardiac endurance. Balance requires input from vision, proprioception, and the vestibular system [32]. PT and OT work together to best meet mobility needs of people with NMD.

Ambulation PT's role is to assess for ways to optimize gait efficiency, speed, and balance. This aids individuals in energy management, safety, and fall prevention while walking. When people with NMD present with impairments in strength, endurance, range of motion, sensation, or their balance system, they may need an assistive device (AD) and/or an orthotic to compensate for these changes and improve safety and efficiency with walking. Strengthening is not always the first or best approach with this population.

Commonly used ADs include canes, walking poles, forearm crutches, and walkers. A walker may have no wheels, two front wheels, or four wheels with a seat and brakes. Generally a cane with a single point has less support than a walker with four legs.

There are many factors involved in determining the most appropriate assistive device for ambulation. These include a person's acceptance of the device, the degree of physical impairment, the functional mobility distance required at home and in the community, and the rate of disease progression. A person with ALS and rapidly progressive postural decline, declining respiratory function, and lower extremity weakness may benefit from a four-wheeled walker. This would be based in part on

Table 7.3 Validated assessments performed by therapists in people with NMD
Assessments in red test impairment and assessments in blue test activity limitations

IMPAIRMENT	INSTRUMENT	ASSESSED BY
Range of motion	Goniometry	PT, OT or hand therapist
Distal upper limb strength	Dynamometry (lateral pinch, palmar pinch, grip)	OT or hand therapist
Strength	Manual Muscle Testing (MMT)	PT, OT or hand therapy
Proximal lower limb strength	5-times sit to stand [7]	PT
Gross motor coordination	Box and Blocks Test [8] Alternating Foot Tap Test	PT or OT
Fine motor coordination	NineHole Peg Test [9]	OT or hand therapist
Mobility and gait	Timed Up and Go (TUG) [10] 6-Minute Timed Walk (6MTW) [44] Timed 25 Foot Walk (T25-FW) [11] Dynamic Gait Index (DGI) [12] (Modified) Clinical Test of Sensory Interaction and Balance (CTSIB/mCTSIB) [13] Functional Gait Assessment (FGA) [45] Romberg Test Single Limb Stance (SLS) [14]	PT
Spasticity	Modified Ashworth scale [15]	PT or OT
Balance	Berg Balance Scale (BBS) [16]	PT
Sensation	Semmes-Weinstein monofilament	PT or OT
Vision	Brain Injury Visual Assessment Battery for Adults (biVABA) [46] Dynavision® [47]	OT
Swallowing	Bedside swallow Fiberoptic Endoscopic Evaluation of Swallow (FEES) Video-fluoroscopic Swallow Study (VFSS)	SLP

(continued)

Table 7.3 (continued)

Speech	Speech Intelligibility Test (SIT) [17]	SLP
	Assessment in Intelligibility of Dysarthric Speech (AIDS) [18]	
	Frenchay Dysarthria Assessment 2nd Edition (FDA-2) [19]	
Language	Cognitive Linguistic Quick Test (CLQT) [20]	SLP
	Woodcock Johnson Test of Achievement [48]	
	Repeatable Battery for the Assessment of Neuropsychological Status (RBANS) [21]	
	Minnesota Test for Differential Diagnosis of Aphasia (MTDDA) [49]	
	Boston Diagnostic Aphasia Examination (BDAE) [22]	
	Boston Naming Test (BNT) [22]	
	Western Aphasia Battery (WAB) [23]	
Cognition and behavior	Montreal Cognitive Assessment (MOCA) [24]	OT or SLP
	Frontal Systems Behavioral Scale (FrSBe) [25, 26]	
	ALS Cognitive Behavioral Screen (ALS-CBS) [27]	
	Edinburgh Cognitive Assessment Screen (ECAS) [28]	
	Cognitive Performance Test (CPT) [29]	
Fatigue	Modified Fatigue Impact Scale [30]	OT or PT
	Fatigue Severity Scale [31]	

knowledge that further functional decline may be expected by their next 3- or 6-month follow-up visit and that it will provide the best postural support and allow for seated rest breaks with mobility. By contrast, a person with only foot drop and mild imbalance from CMT, with an anticipated slower progression of weakness, may need only an ankle-foot orthosis with a cane or walking poles to provide adequate support for a longer period of time.

In addition to determining which AD may optimize safe ambulation, PTs and OTs consider other factors that may influence use, such as use of the device to aid other aspects of ADLs and IADLs. For example, a four-wheeled walker with a seat may best allow a person to sit at the bathroom sink to reduce fatigue while grooming or to allow for safe transport of supplies, such as with meal preparation or laundry.

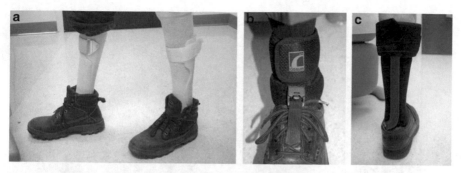

Fig. 7.1 Plastic AFO, Foot-Up® brace, and carbon fiber AFO

Given the costs and insurance limitations for AD payment, PTs must also predict which AD will serve the person for the longest period of time to meet his or her needs for safe and effective ambulation.

Lower extremity orthoses There is a variety of lower extremity supports that can be beneficial separately or in conjunction with an AD. These include a knee support, an ankle-foot orthosis (AFO), or other less restrictive ankle supports to aid in stability and alleviate foot drop. This is best determined by a PT in conjunction with an orthotist. An orthotist will fabricate and fit a custom AFO if a prefabricated AFO or ankle brace is inadequate to meet a person's needs. Examples of prefabricated ankle supports include the Ossur Foot-Up Drop Foot Brace® and lightweight plastic and carbon fiber AFOs (Fig. 7.1).

Seating and wheeled mobility When functional ambulation is limited by respiratory decline, weakness, or impaired endurance and balance, it may be time for a person to pursue an alternative means of mobility with the help of their PT or OT. Wheeled mobility devices include manual or powered wheelchairs and scooters. Decisions about which is the most appropriate device are determined by the accessibility of the person's home, cognitive and physical status for safe operation, methods to transport it, level of caregiver support, and willingness to accept an alternative means of mobility. These devices may augment or replace ambulation when they are needed for safe and effective mobility. Disease type is paramount in determining if a person will have the upper body strength, range of motion, endurance, and balance to operate a manual wheelchair or if they will benefit from pursuing powered mobility.

Both manual and powered wheelchairs allow for custom seating and positioning. Depending upon individual needs and extent of weakness, a person with NMD may require a pressure-relieving or custom cushion and supports for the foot, thigh, back, trunk, arm, head, or neck. Positioning options include tilt-in-space, recline, elevated foot rests, seat elevator, and standing ability. These methods are used to provide pressure relief and pressure sore prevention, position change for comfort, edema reduction, stretching and weight bearing, and assistance with transfers (Figs. 7.2, 7.3, 7.4, and 7.5).

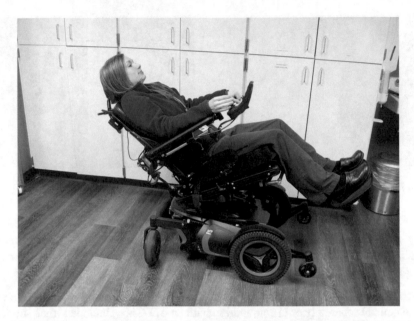

Fig. 7.2 Tilt-in-space option on front-wheel drive Permobil F5 power wheelchair™

Fig. 7.3 Standing

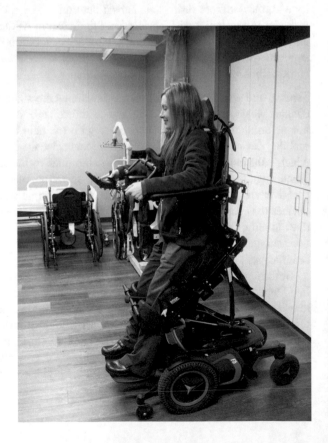

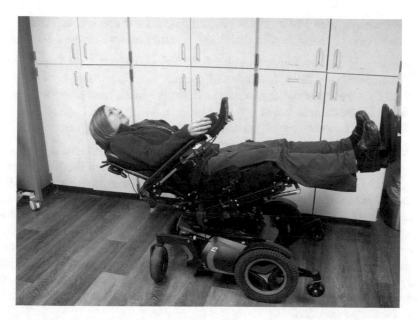

Fig. 7.4 Recline and foot elevation

Fig. 7.5 Seat elevation

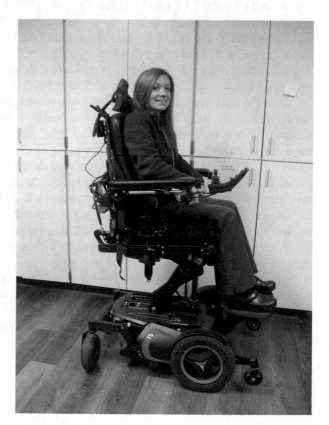

Some people with NMD do not have sufficient hand strength and dexterity to operate a power wheelchair with their hand. Alternatives include the following:

- Joysticks of various shapes (straight, ball, domed, u-shaped, etc.) or touchpads allow operation of the wheelchair with a hand.
- Head array and other switch control operations use subtle head or extremity movement with pressure switches.
- Sip-and-puff control: breath pressure is translated into driving control.

An assistive technology practitioner (ATP) is a therapy clinician or equipment supplier who has undergone training and certification through the Rehabilitation Engineering and Assistive Technology Society of North America (RESNA) to assess the needs of people with disabilities for assistive technology, identify technologies that are appropriate, and train them in their use [33]. The use of a scooter or a powered wheelchair is best determined by an OT or PT who is also credentialed as an ATP. PTs and OTs specializing in this field are able to stay up to date on current insurance coverage guidelines, technology for operation, and seating and positioning options. This is critical in determining the most appropriate seating and wheeled mobility device based on current level of function and projected function with disease progression.

Functional transfers OTs and PTs both provide critical input to optimize safety with functional transfers, including moving to and from a bed, chair, wheelchair, or toilet, stepping in and out of a tub or shower, and getting in and out of a vehicle. There are many types of equipment to help people with transfers from one surface to another and from a sitting to standing position. For example, someone with inclusion body myositis (IBM) may have difficulty rising from lower surfaces due to proximal lower body weakness. Adaptations in this case include furniture risers, a dense foam cushion on furniture to increase height, a power lift recliner chair, a raised toilet seat with handles, or a powered toilet seat lift. Other individuals may have optimized home accessibility but still benefit from training a caregiver to provide light support by lifting with a transfer belt to help the person rise from a chair. A person with proximal and distal lower extremity weakness from ALS may need an extended tub transfer bench and training by an OT to allow for a seated transfer in and out of the tub when they can no longer step over the side of the tub. Other equipment may include a bed rail to help with moving from lying to sitting or a floor to ceiling pole to aid in moving from sitting to standing where grab bars cannot be installed.

Training includes teaching caregivers and people with NMD to avoid injuries. Such injuries may occur by pulling on a weakened arm or lifting a person's entire weight. Some medical institutional standards have suggested lifting no greater than 35 pounds for injury prevention [34]. OTs and PTs assess people with NMD for weakness to determine when mechanical lifting devices are needed for caregiver and client safety and fall prevention.

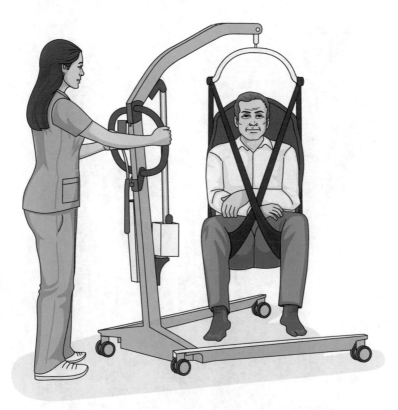

Fig. 7.6 Manual lift

Mechanical lifting devices include a standing lift system or a non-weight-bearing sling lift system (Figs. 7.6 and 7.7). Standing lift systems allow for weight bearing with legs and feet on a platform with a sling support behind one's back in order to manually lift and pivot to an adjacent surface. For a weaker person without lower extremity weight-bearing capacity, a mechanical lift with a sling and a wheeled base may be required. These can also be used to assist a person up from a fall to the floor. There are also ceiling lift systems using a sling. This may ease transfers from a bed to a wheelchair or to a toilet in another room.

Standing frames and standing features on power wheelchairs also aid mobility (Fig. 7.8). These prevent contractures and pressure sores, improve bowel and bladder function, maintain bone density and postural reflexes, and in some cases maintain strength of lower extremities and postural muscles [35].

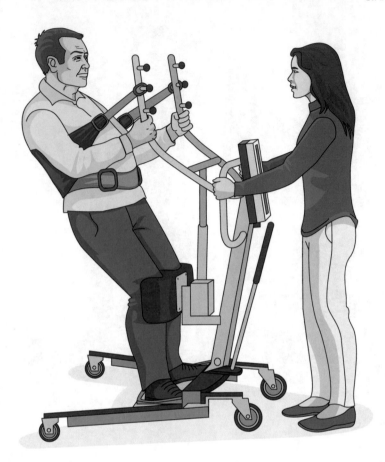

Fig. 7.7 Standing lift

Home Accessibility

OT and PT assessment and training for home accessibility is a key component of help-ing people with NMD plan for disease progression and optimize their quality of life. Early planning is needed for people with anticipated progressive disability, as remodel-ing is expensive and takes time. Simple adaptations may include a swing clear door hinge adaptation to allow for a wider doorway to accommodate a wheelchair or walker, a stair lift to allow a person to safely move from one level of the home to another, or a threshold ramp to allow access across a threshold in and out of the home. More com-plex planning is needed when a person anticipates the need for a manual or power wheelchair, a wheeled shower commode chair, or a manual lift device. This may include remodeling for main level living, a roll-in barrier free shower, or a ramp to enter the home. If main level living is not possible, a stair lift, wheelchair platform lift, or an elevator to move between levels may be needed. OTs and PTs may work directly with contractors or educate people with NMD about the importance of working with home contractors or other professionals who specialize in home accessibility.

Fig. 7.8 Standing frame

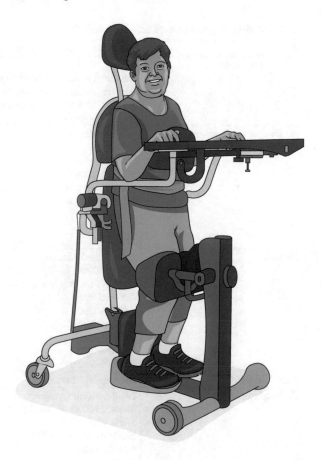

ADL/IADL, EADL, Adaptive Equipment, and Upper Body Orthoses

ADL/IADL and adaptive equipment OTs assess a person's limitations in ADLs and IADLs and identify solutions. Therapists analyze daily living activities that are meaningful to a person in order to break the tasks down into manageable parts, so they can complete them with modifications. Table 7.4 lists examples of adapted techniques and adaptive equipment available to complete ADLs and IADLs.

In addition to identifying specific adaptations, therapists also identify options for energy conservation in consideration of the fatigue associated with most NMDs. For example, they may recommend caregiver assistance with dressing so that the person with NMD is able to conserve energy for tasks that they find most meaningful.

In some cases, therapists can administer functional scales that serve both to identify a patient's therapy needs and act as a validated measure of disease progression.

Table 7.4 Adaptations to complete ADLs and IADLs

ADL	Examples of adaptations and equipment
Dressing upper body	Looser clothing Lie down to don overhead shirts Weaker arm in first and out last Adapted fasteners (magnetic or Velcro shirt front) Button hook aid
Dressing lower body	Long shoehorn Sock aid Reacher Slip-on shoes Elastic shoelaces Elastic waist pants Suspenders Zipper pull Sit for task
Feeding	Larger-handled utensils Universal cuff to slip utensils into Nose cut out cup to aid safe swallow Covered mug Scoop plate Rocker knife Wrist brace Elbow support Bestic® feeder
Tube feedings	Feeding tube holders
Bathing/showering	Long-handled sponge Shower seat or wheeled shower commode Wash mitt Handheld shower nozzle Nonslip mat Grab bars
Toileting	Raised toilet or toilet seat Grab bars Bidets Long-handled wiping aids
Brushing teeth	Built-up foam on toothbrush handle Electric toothbrush Automatic toothpaste dispensers
Shaving	Electric razors Built-up foam on razor handle Sit to prop arms
Styling hair	Long-handled brushes and combs Hair dryer mounts Sit to prop arms to reach the head
Washing hair	Long-handled hair washers Sit to prop arms to reach the head
IADL	Examples of adaptations and equipment

(continued)

Table 7.4 (continued)

ADL	Examples of adaptations and equipment
Writing for communication	Built-up pen grips PenAgain® Wanchik Writer®
Typing for communication	Typing aid Voice dictation software or voice-to-text features Clamp-on forearm supports Figure-of-eight finger supports
Phone use	Voice-activated phone Switch-activated phone Bluetooth switch
Wash dishes	Sit on tall stool at sink Light dishware
Oven use	Sit on stool; oven rack push/pull Lighter-weight dishware
Shopping	Powered scooter or wheelchair Online shopping Grocery delivery Wheeled grocery carriers
Meal preparation	Wheeled cart or four-wheeled walker to transport items Adapted knives to cut Lower microwave to counter top level Toaster oven
Financial management	Writing aids Online and auto-pay options
Gardening/yard care	Adapted gardening tools Hydraulic hose winders Self-propel lawn mower or riding mower Hired help
Child care	Adapted cribs and changing tables
Driving	Adapted driving equipment such as hand controls Left gas pedal extension Gravity-reduced steering Key holders

An example of such an assessment is the ALS Functional Rating Scale-Revised (ALSFRS-R), a self-report measure of ADLs, mobility, swallowing, communication, and ventilatory function [36].

EADL and assistive technology People with NMD have access to a vast array of ever-changing assistive technology to assist with environmental access. Examples of EADLs are listed in Table 7.5.

Upper body orthoses People with NMD benefit from many types of upper body supports, such as hand splints and neck braces. OTs, hand therapists, PTs, and orthotists are consulted to help with assessment and fitting of these devices. Table 7.6 lists examples of upper body orthoses for people with NMD.

Table 7.5 Examples of EADLs

Environmental need	EADL/assistive technology options
Electronic control of appliances such as TV, fan, and lights	Wemo® by Belkin or other appliance modules that are Wi-Fi enabled using smartphone or tablet to activate electronic devices such as TV, fan, and lights Switch-adapted appliance and light modules with remotes Voice-activated environmental controller Use of power wheelchair electronics to control appliances via joystick, pressure switches, or sip-and-puff
Call light	Adapted pressure switch placed on the head, extremity, or mouth or sip-and-puff switch
Door opening	Adapted pressure switches to activate electric door opener Lever handles Key holders
Computer access	Voice recognition software Text-to-speech apps Head dot mouse with wireless optical sensor Eye tracking technology Adapted mouse such as joystick style with thumb control or rollerball style

Table 7.6 Examples of upper body orthoses for people with NMD

Problem	Orthosis
Claw hand from intrinsic weakness	Metacarpophalangeal (MCP) joint extension block splint to allow finger extension
Weak palmar thumb pinch	Prefabricated thumb support or custom palmar abduction thumb splint
Weak finger extension	Neoprene finger sleeve or figure-of-eight splint over PIP joint
Finger flexor tightness from spasticity or finger extensor weakness	Forearm to finger custom resting hand splint
Tremor, wrist extensor weakness, or median nerve irritation	Prefabricated wrist cock-up brace or custom wrist cock-up splint
Shoulder glenohumeral subluxation	Prefabricated hemi-shoulder supports Wheelchair arm trough/support
Neck weakness	Soft foam collar Headmaster collar® Ballert Oxford Collar® Rigid collar
Neck extensor weakness and dysphagia	Ballert Oxford Collar®
Truncal weakness	Prefabricated or custom made trunk/back supports

Functional Vision

Several neuromuscular conditions such as myasthenia gravis, mitochondrial disorders, myotonic dystrophy, and oculopharyngeal muscular dystrophy can result in functional visual loss due to ptosis, oculomotor weakness, or cataracts [37]. Functionally, this can impact reading, ADLs, IADLs, and mobility. OTs can help with adaptations such as improved lighting, increased contrast such as bright tape on a stair edge, or use of enlarged print. When indicated, optometrists can recommend eye masks at night, lubrication drops, surgery, an eyeglass ptosis crutch, patching, or prisms for functional visual impairments (Fig. 7.9).

Fatigue and Impaired Respiratory and Cardiac Function

Many forms of NMD are associated with respiratory or cardiac compromise. It is important for PT, OT, and SLP clinicians to be aware of respiratory or cardiac impairments that may limit safety or tolerance of activity. Mobility aids and energy conservation measures may be needed in such patients despite relatively functional muscle strength (Table 7.7).

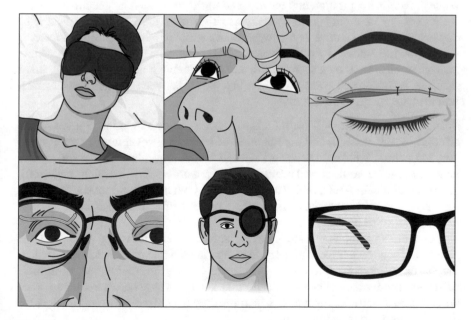

Fig. 7.9 Optometry interventions to improve functional vision

Table 7.7 Examples of function impacted by compromised respiratory or cardiac status

Example	Energy management strategies
Fatigue with eating	Use of noninvasive ventilation (NIV) prior to, partway through, or following mealtimes
Fatigue with ADL	Pacing, doing task in parts, frequent rests, sitting for tasks, use of adaptive equipment, avoid bending, and use of NIV before, during, or following ADL
Fatigue with mobility	Use of a powered wheelchair or assistive device for mobility

Swallowing, Speech, and Augmentative and Alternative Communication (AAC)

Swallowing and dysphagia SLPs are responsible for assessing swallowing function. The jaw, lips, tongue, and pharyngeal musculature move food, drinks, and secretions into the esophagus and protect the airway from aspiration [38]. Weakness in any or all of these muscle groups can lead to impaired swallowing or poor management of saliva. Swallow function can be assessed through clinical observation or more objectively with a videofluoroscopic swallow study (VFSS) or fiberoptic endoscopic evaluation of swallow (FEES) (Fig. 7.10). Based on evaluation results, recommendations can be made for diet modifications and/or swallowing strategies to increase ease and safety of swallowing. The ultimate goal is to ensure nutrition while preventing aspiration and resulting complications such as pneumonia. SLPs work closely with dieticians to optimize nutrition when diet restrictions need to be implemented and to reduce energy expenditure while maximizing caloric intake.

Swallowing safety is also impacted by respiratory status. Those who cannot manage or clear their own secretions due to a weak cough may need a cough assist machine, which provides a rapid change in pressure between inhalation and exhalation to make cough more effective.

Speech and Dysarthria Dysarthria is a change in speech function. Speech can be affected by the strength and coordination of breathing, vocal cords, tongue, lips, jaw, and velum. Weakness of the cranial and bulbar musculature occurs in several neuromuscular conditions and results in impaired articulation, nasal air emissions, and hypophonia. In ALS a mixed dysarthria with both flaccid and spastic features is most common, with elements of weakness, slow and effortful speech, and a strained or strangled voice quality.

SLP clinicians implement strategies to improve intelligibility and reduce fatigue. Strategies focus on compensations such as slowing the rate of speech, overarticulating, facing the person one is speaking to, and changing the environment to promote easier and more efficient communication. The diagnosis dictates whether a person will develop dysarthria, the type of dysarthria they may experience, and whether the dysarthria will progress to anarthria.

Dysphonia Some patients with NMD experience weakness or paralysis in the muscles responsible for movements of the vocal cords. This may, in turn, result in a

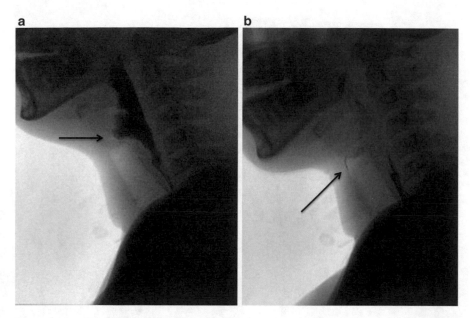

Fig. 7.10 (**a**) Penetration: swallowed contents enter the airway but remain above the vocal folds. (**b**) Aspiration: swallowed material is below the vocal folds and enters the anterior aspect of the trachea

disorder of the sound of speech called dysphonia. At times, voice therapy can help improve the use of the affected muscles.

Augmentative and Alternative Communication Augmentative and alternative communication (AAC) is used to supplement or replace verbal communication. For those who are hypophonic but able to speak intelligibly, a voice amplifier alone may be sufficient to allow effective communication. For those who cannot communicate verbally but have preserved upper limb functional movement and want a simple means of communication, writing on a notepad, dry erase board, or Boogie Board® LCD Writing Tablet (which erases quickly) (Fig. 7.11) may suffice for communication. Others with more severe impairment can point to letters or symbols on a communication board with eyes or limbs to make needs known [38] or simply blink and move the eyes or head at a certain frequency to communicate yes/no and other basic needs.

In many instances, a computer, tablet, or smartphone may be used as an AAC. Different computer devices have different options for accessibility. Computer use may involve voice output software on a PC or a specific speech-generating device. Mobile devices such as smartphones and tablets can be used with voice output applications. Many devices can be accessed by switches that scan and select on-screen data with small movements of the hand, head, and limb.

A computer may also be mounted and accessed with the use of head dot or eye gaze technology (Figs. 7.12 and 7.13). A head dot pointer involves placement of a quarter-inch-sized reflective dot placed on a body part (typically the forehead), monitored by a camera above the screen, to select items with an on-screen mouse and

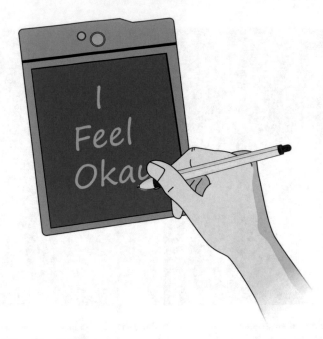

Fig. 7.11 LCD writing tablet

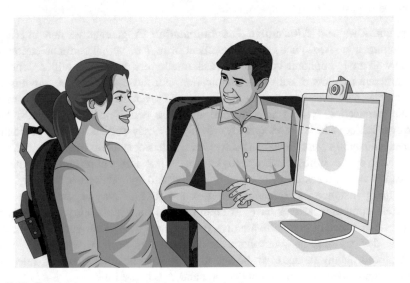

Fig. 7.12 Computer access with head dot mouse technology

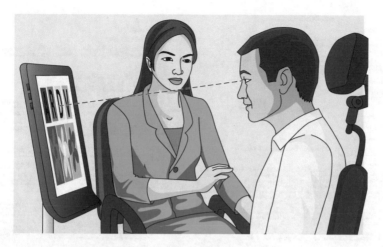

Fig. 7.13 Speech generating device used with eye tracking technology

keyboard. Eye gaze technology allows similar access but with eye movements detected by infrared light reflecting off the retina. Devices usually implement word prediction to improve speed of communication.

Cognition and Behavior

Cognitive and behavioral changes are common in people with some neuromuscular diseases. For example, up to 50% of people with ALS demonstrate some degree of cognitive and/or behavioral impairment, and a small proportion develop frontotemporal dementia [39]. Myotonic dystrophy is also commonly associated with cognitive dysfunction [40]. It is important to screen cognition and behavior early in the course of disease and as it progresses, as safety, communication effectiveness, medical decision-making, and the need for caregiver support can all be affected. People with NMD also need to learn to use equipment, such as walkers and power wheelchairs. It is important to assure that people with NMD have not only the physical means to complete a task but also the cognitive capability to do so safely.

Many assessments can be used to screen cognitive and behavioral function. The ALS Cognitive Behavioral Screen (ALS-CBS) may be used to screen for both cognitive and behavioral impairments in ALS [39]. Screening instruments may be completed by many different members of a multidisciplinary care team such as an OT, SLP, or nurse. If impairment is suspected, more comprehensive evaluation by a neuropsychologist to define degree and type of impairment as well as the influence of mental health on current level of functioning may be warranted.

Therapists can also assess the functional impacts of cognitive deficits on IADLs and safety. One such assessment performed by occupational therapists is the cognitive performance test (CPT), which assesses functional cognitive disability (Fig. 7.14) [41]. The CPT helps to make recommendations regarding the level of living support

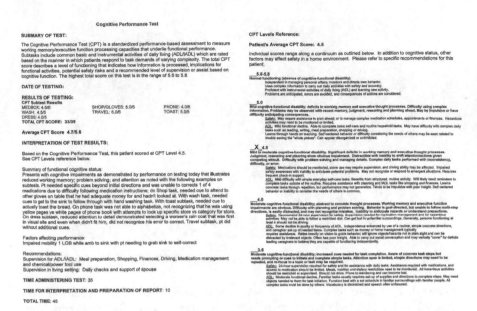

Fig. 7.14 Example of a Cognitive Performance Test (CPT) report

one may require, methods to help the person and family compensate, work ability, or driving risk, for example. SLPs also have numerous assessments to assess for functional cognitive and language (comprehension and expression) deficits as well.

Exercise, Spasticity Management, and Contracture Prevention

Exercise Some people with NMDs hope to stop or slow progression of their disease process by exercising. Exercise prescription needs to be undertaken with caution by skilled PTs, OTs, and SLPs aware of current research implications for exercise based on the type and progression of disease, acuity of the condition, and the form of exercise implicated. Two common forms of exercise are aerobic conditioning and strengthening.

Aerobic, or cardiovascular, exercise involves activities such as walking, cycling, and other means of exercising to build cardiac, respiratory, and muscle endurance. For many forms of NMD, aerobic exercise is an important component of disease management, with benefits beyond fitness such as improved digestion, mood, and bone density. For instance, for a person diagnosed with CMT, aerobic conditioning that maintains proximal and truncal strength can promote improved function over time to compensate for distal weakness. Moderate exercise has been shown to be beneficial in slowly progressive muscular dystrophies [42]. Low- or moderate-intensity aerobic exercise may be of benefit for people living with ALS [43]. Pool exercise is particularly valuable for cardiovascular health, endurance, and strengthening in patients who have imbalance or ankle instability from NMD. Therapy clinicians need to be aware of their patients' current cardiac and respiratory status, strength, and baseline activity level and fitness to help them make the best choices regarding the level and type of aerobic conditioning indicated.

Strengthening or resistance training needs to be undertaken with care as well, as it may have adverse or potentially beneficial effects in NMD [42, 43]. In addition clinicians need to consider the effects of inactivity, as muscle atrophy from disuse may occur in addition to that caused by disease and, in turn, affect mobility and quality of life. People with NMD should monitor themselves closely during and after exercise for symptoms such as fatigue, muscle cramps and pain, increase in weakness, or pigmenturia as a sign of muscle destruction [42]. Cardiology consultation may be required prior to designing an exercise regimen for people with NMDs affecting cardiac muscle or conduction [42].

Spasticity management and contracture prevention Stretching and training in assisted or passive range of motion are appropriate in many instances and in most diagnoses of NMD where weakness and/or spasticity is present and can delay or reduce the need for pharmacologic interventions to manage spasticity. This helps prevent muscle and joint contracture and immobility that can lead to pain, difficulty completing ADLs, and reduced functional use of a limb. Caregiver training to help those who lack the physical strength or means to complete their own range of motion is important, as range of motion exercise can be fatiguing for some. Orthotics also aid in positioning and preventing joint contractures.

Summary

PT, OT, and SLP clinicians are an integral part of a multidisciplinary team helping people with NMDs live functional and meaningful lives. There are many ways to address functional impairments associated with these conditions. It is important to assess people regularly over their disease course to provide appropriate interventions for their changing functional abilities based on their diagnosis and disease progression.

Acknowledgments Special thanks to Karen Stine, MS, CCC-SLP; Sara Junge, MS, CCC-SLP; Cynthia Gackle OTR/L; Monica Wainio, PT; and Jackie Geiser, PT, DPT for their invaluable contributions to this chapter.

References

1. World Health Organization. Towards a Common Language for Functioning, Disability and Health: ICF [Internet]. 2002 [cited 2017 February 19]. Available from: http://www.who.int/classifications/icf/icfbeginnersguide.pdf?ua=1.
2. American Occupational Therapy Association. Scope of practice. Am J Occup Ther. 2014;68(Suppl 3):S35. https://doi.org/10.5014/ajot.2014.686S04.
3. American Physical Therapy Association. The physical therapist scope of practice [Internet]. 2015 [updated 2015 Nov 20; cited 2016 Oct 12]:1. Available from: http://www.apta.org/ScopeOfPractice/.

4. American Speech-Language-Hearing Association. Scope of practice in speech-language pathology [Internet]. 2016 [updated 2016 Feb 4; cited 2016 Oct 12]:2. Available from: http://www.asha.org/policy/SP2016-00343/.
5. American Board for Certification in Orthotics, Prosthetics, and Pedorthics [Internet]. 2017 [cited 2017 Feb 20]. Available from: https://www.abcop.org/individual-certification/Pages/orthotistandprosthetist.aspx.
6. American Society of Hand Therapists [Internet]. 2017 [cited 2017 Feb 20]. Available from: https://www.asht.org/patients.
7. Whitney L, Wrisley M, Marchetti F, Gee A, Redfern S, Furman M. Clinical measurement of sit-to-stand performance in people with balance disorders: validity of data for the Five-Times-Sit-to-Stand-Test. Phys Ther. 2005;85(10):1034–45.
8. Mathiowetz V, Volland G, Kashman N, Weber K. Adult norms for the box and blocks test of manual dexterity. Am J Occup Ther. 1985;39:389–91.
9. Mathiowetz V, Weber K, Kashman N, Volland G. Adult norms for the Nine Hole Peg Test of finger dexterity. Occup Ther J Res. 1985;5:24–38.
10. Podsiadlo D, Richardson S. The timed "Up & Go": a test of basic functional mobility for frail elderly persons. J Am Geriatr Soc. 1991;39:142–8.
11. Motl R, Cohen J, Benedict R, Phillips G, LaRocca N, et al. Validity of the timed 25-foot walk as an ambulatory performance outcome measure for multiple sclerosis. Mult Scler. 2017;23:704–10.
12. Shumway-Cook A, Woollacott M. Motor control: theory and applications. Wilkins & Wilkins: Baltimore; 1995.
13. Shumway-Cook A, Horak FB. Assessing the influence of sensory interaction on balance. Phys Ther. 1986;66:1548–50.
14. Bohannon R. Single Limb Stance times a descriptive Meta-Analysis of data from individuals at least 60 years of age. Top Geriatr Rehabil. 2006;22:70–7.
15. Ashworth B. Preliminary trial of carisoprodol in multiple sclerosis. Practitioner. 1964;192:540–2.
16. Berg K, Wood-Dauphine S, Williams JI, Gayton D. Measuring balance in the elderly: preliminary development of an instrument. Physiother Can. 1989;41:304–11.
17. Yorkston KM, Beukemam DR. Communication efficiency of dysarthric speakers as measured by sentence intelligibility and speaking rate. J Speech Hear Disord. 1981;46:296–301.
18. Yorkston KM, Beukelman DR. Assessment of intelligibility of dysarthric speech. Austin: Pro-Ed; 1984.
19. Enderby P, Palmer R. Frenchay dysarthria assessment–Second edition. Austin: Pro-Ed; 2008.
20. Helm-Estabrooks N. Cognitive Linguistic Quick Test (CLQT): Examiner's Manual.
21. Randolph C, Tierney MC, Mohr E, Chase TN. The repeatable battery for the assessment of neuropsychological status (RBANS): preliminary clinical validity. Clin Exp Neuropsychol. 1998;20:310–9.
22. Goodglass H, Kaplan E, Baressi B. Boston Diagnostic Aphasia Examination: Short form record booklet. 3rd ed. Boston: Lippincott, Williams, & Wilkins; 2001.
23. Shewan CM, Kertesz A. Reliability and validity characteristics of the Western aphasia battery (WAB). J Speech Hear Disord. 1980;45:308–24.
24. Nasreddine ZS, Philips NA, Bedirian V. The Montreal Cognitive Assessment, MoCA: A brief screening tool for mild cognitive impairment. J Am Geriatr Soc. 2005;52:695–9.
25. Grace J, Stout JC, Malloy PF. Assessing frontal lobe behavioral syndromes with the Frontal Lobe Personality Scale. Assessment. 1999;6:269–84.
26. Grace J, Malloy PF. Frontal Systems Behavior Scale (FrSBe): Professional Manual. Lutz: Psychological Assessment Resources; 2001.
27. Wooley SE, York M, Moore D, Strutt A, Murphy J. Detecting frontotemporal dementia in ALS: utility of the ALS cognitive behavioral screen (ALS-CBS). ALS. 2010;11:303.
28. Abrahams S, Newton J, Niven E, Foley J, Bak T. Screening for cognition and behavior changes in ALS. ALS-FTD. 2014;15:9–14.
29. Burns T. Cognitive performance test manual. Maddak: Pequannock; 2006.
30. Ritvo PG, Fischer JS, Miller DM, Andrews H, Paty DW, LaRocca NG. MSQLI: Multiple Sclerosis Quality of Life Inventory: A User's Manual. New York: National Multiple Sclerosis Society; 1997.

31. Krupp LB. The fatigue severity scale. Application to patients with multiple sclerosis and systemic lupus erythematosus. Arch Neurol. 1989;46:1121–3.
32. Vestibular Disorders Association. The human balance system [Internet]. 2016 [cited 2016 Oct 12]:1. Available from: http://vestibular.org/understanding-vestibular-disorder/human-balance-system.
33. Rehabilitation Engineering and Assistive Technology Society of North America (RESNA). Assistive technology practitioner certification [Internet]. 2015 [cited 2016 Oct 12]: 1. Available from: http://www.resna.org/get-certified/atp/atp-0.
34. Centers for Disease Control and Prevention. The National Institute for Occupational Safety and Health. Safe patient handling and movement [Internet]. 2016 [updated 2016 July 22; cited 2016 Oct 12]:1. Available from: https://www.cdc.gov/niosh/topics/safepatient/.
35. Wechsler K. Stand up and go with mobile standers and standing wheelchairs [Internet]. Quest MDA's Research and Health Magazine. 2011 Jan 1 [cited 2016 Oct 12]:1. Available from: http://quest.mda.org/article/stand-and-go-mobile-standers-and-standing-wheelchairs.
36. Cedarbaum J, Stambler N, Malta E, Fuller C, Hilt D, Thurmond B, Nakanishi A. The ALSFRS-R: a revised ALS functional rating scale that incorporates assessments of respiratory function. J Neurol Sci. 1999;169(1–2):13–21.
37. Wahl M. Keeping your focus: Eye care in neuromuscular disorders. Quest MDA's Research and Health Magazine. 2000 Dec 1 [cited 2016 Jun 15]. Available from: http://quest.mda.org/article/keeping-your-focus-eye-care.
38. Carr-Davis E, Blakely-Adams C, Corinblit B. Living with ALS, adjusting to swallowing and speaking difficulties. The ALS Association: Calabasas Hills, CA; 2007.
39. Woolley S, York M, Moore A, Strutt A, Murphy J, Schulz P, Katz J. Detecting frontotemporal dysfunction in ALS: utility of the ALS cognitive behavioral screen (ALS-CBS). ALS. 2010;11:303–11.
40. Muscular Dystrophy Association. Myotonic muscular dystrophy (MMD). 2016 [cited 2016 Oct 12]. Available from: https://www.mda.org/disease/myotonic-muscular-dystrophy.
41. Burns T. The cognitive performance test (CPT). Manual. 2013;2013:1–4.
42. Muscular Dystrophy Association. Exercising with a muscle disease. Quest MDA's Research and Health Magazine [Internet]. 2009 April 1 [cited 2016 Jun 12]:1–17 Available from: http://quest.mda.org/series/exercising-muscle-disease.
43. Dal Bello-Haas V, Florence J, Kloos A, Scheirbecker J, Lopate G, Hayes S, Pioro E, Mitsumoto H. A randomized controlled trial of resistance exercise in individuals with ALS. Neurol. 2007;68(23):2003–7.
44. Steffen TM, Hacker TA, Mollinger L. Age- and gender-related test performance in community-dwelling elderly people: six-minute walk test, Berg balance scale, timed up and go test, and gait speeds. Phys Ther 2002;82:128–137.
45. Wrisley DM, Marchetti GF, Kuharsky DK, Whitney SL. Reliability, internal consistency, and validity of data obtained with the functional gait assessment. Phys Ther 2004;84:906–918.
46. Warren M. published by visABILITIES Rehab Services Inc., www.visabilities.com
47. products.dynavisioninternational.com
48. Woodcock RW, Mather N, McGrew K. Woodcock-Johnson III tests of achievement. Itasca IL: Riverside, 2001.
49. Schuell H. Differential diagnosis of aphasia with the Minnesota test. Minneapolis: University of Minnesota Press, 1965.

Resources

Muscular Dystrophy Association [Internet]. Available from: https://www.mda.org/.
The ALS Association [Internet]. Available from: https://www.alsa.org.

Chapter 8
Electrodiagnostic Testing

Jeffrey A. Allen

Abbreviations

CMAP	Compound muscle action potential
CRD	Complex repetitive discharges
DRG	Dorsal root ganglion
EMG	Electromyography
Fibs	Fibrillation potentials
MUAP	Motor action unit potential
NCS	Nerve conduction studies
PSW	Positive sharp waves
SNAP	Sensory nerve action potential

Key Points
- A good electrodiagnostic study starts with a specific question and evolves as new information that is uncovered during the test.
- Failure to adequately warm a patient during NCS may result in erroneously slow conduction velocities or prolonged distal latencies.
- Although small motor and sensory amplitudes on NCS typically represent axon loss, other explanations include severe muscle or neuromuscular junction injury, distal conduction block, or submaximal nerve stimulation.
- In conduction block, both amplitude and area are reduced, whereas in temporal dispersion amplitude drops, but area is relatively preserved, and duration is prolonged. Both suggest focal nerve demyelination.
- Sensory responses are measured in µV and motor responses are measured in mV. The smaller sensory responses are technically more challenging to accurately record and require greater attention to detail in order to minimize external electric noise.

J.A. Allen (✉)
University of Minnesota Medical Center, Department of Neurology, Minneapolis, MN, USA
e-mail: jaallen@UMN.edu

© Springer International Publishing AG, part of Springer Nature 2018
D. Walk (ed.), *Clinical Handbook of Neuromuscular Medicine*,
https://doi.org/10.1007/978-3-319-67116-1_8

- Late response abnormalities are not specific for proximal nerve injury, but if distal recordings are normal and late responses are abnormal, the presumption is that the lesion is localized to a proximal segment.
- Dorsal nerve root lesions proximal to the dorsal root ganglion may cause sensory symptoms but have normal sensory nerve conduction studies.
- NCS assess large motor and sensory fibers. Polyneuropathies that affect only small fibers (small fiber polyneuropathy) may have normal nerve conduction studies.
- Reduced amplitude NCS usually indicate axon loss. Slow CV, prolonged latency, CB, and temporal dispersion usually indicate demyelination.
- Referencing available electrodiagnostic demyelinating guidelines can provide clarity when amplitude reductions and CV slowing are both present in a single nerve.
- End plate noise and spikes are normal and should not be confused with other pathologic forms of spontaneous activity
- Fibrillation potentials and positive sharp waves can be seen with both neurogenic and myopathic disorders that result in denervation or muscle membrane instability.
- Fasciculation potentials may be normal, benign, or part of a peripheral nerve disorder but are not seen in primary myopathic conditions.
- Large, long, polyphasic MUAPs are classically seen in chronic neurogenic disorders.
- Short, brief, polyphasic MUAPs are classically seen in myopathies.
- Reduced recruitment – neurogenic
- Early recruitment – myopathic

Introduction

Electrodiagnostic testing (nerve conduction studies (NCS) and electromyography (EMG)) is an essential neuromuscular tool [1]. Often called "an extension of the physical exam," NCS/EMG can help clinicians localize lesions, characterize pathophysiology, understand injury severity, and assess chronicity. The intent of this chapter is to highlight abnormalities encountered during routine electrodiagnostic testing and provide the clinician with a framework for how the findings might be interpreted.

Nerve Conduction Studies/Electromyography: Overview

A typical NCS/EMG study starts with a question. Often the referring provider will raise concern over a particular condition, e.g., neuropathy or ALS (Table 8.1). The electrodiagnostic physician uses this referral information and integrates it with a focused clinical history and physical examination taken at the time of the study.

Table 8.1 Common referral questions encountered during NCS/EMG testing

Localization	Disorder
Myopathy	Inflammatory myopathy
	Muscular dystrophy
	Muscle channelopathy
Neuromuscular junction	Myasthenia gravis
	Lambert-Eaton myasthenic syndrome
Focal neuropathies	Median nerve at the wrist
	Ulnar nerve at the elbow
	Peroneal nerve at the knee
Polyneuropathy	Length-dependent polyneuropathy
	Generalized polyneuropathy
	Mononeuropathy multiplex
	Sensory ganglionopathy
Nerve root	Cervical radiculopathy
	Lumbosacral radiculopathy
Plexopathy	Brachial plexopathy
	Lumbosacral plexopathy
Anterior horn cell	Amyotrophic lateral sclerosis
	Spinal muscular atrophy

This information is critical when determining the most appropriate nerves and muscles to be tested. NCS/EMG is a dynamic evaluation. Once the study begins, the choice of nerves and muscles tested evolves based upon the clinical question and in response to electrodiagnostic findings as they emerge [2].

Nerve Conduction Studies

The integrity of the peripheral nervous system can be explored with nerve conduction studies. Surface stimulation of a nerve with a small electrical impulse results in nerve depolarization, action potential generation, and propagation of action potentials in two directions from the point of stimulation. Recordings can then be made of the amplitude and latency of either action potential as it passes beneath a surface recording electrode. In the case of motor conduction studies, recordings can be made of the electrical activity generated by depolarization of muscle cells innervated by the stimulated nerve. Results of the NCS reflect the integrity and function of the myelin sheath and the axon.

Each patient evaluation may include the following recorded NCS responses:

- Motor
- Sensory
- Late responses (F wave and H reflex)

Nerve Conduction Study Procedures

Before the testing begins, the clinician should ensure that the examination room is clean, all supplies needed for the examination are readily available, and the patient is counseled on the procedures anticipated during the test. Temperature of the patient's hand, foot, or other involved areas should be recorded with a goal temperature of ≥ 32 °C in the upper extremity and ≥ 31 °C in the lower extremity. If needed, warming can be performed by submerging the affected limb in a warm water bath. *Inadequate warming will result in artifactually slow conduction velocities and a misdiagnosis of neuropathy* [3].

Electrodes are placed on the skin to record the response from a desired nerve. Electrical stimulation is delivered to the nerve so that the response can be recorded by the electrodes (Fig. 8.1). Current is initially provided at low submaximal levels (5 mA or less) and slowly increased until supramaximal stimulation is achieved, that is, until the amplitude of the response no longer increases with increases in stimulus intensity, indicating that all axons available have been depolarized. The number of stimuli should be minimized when possible. Evoked responses can be measured for latency, amplitude, duration, and conduction velocity (Table 8.2; Fig. 8.2).

Motor Nerve Conduction Studies

Motor NCS are performed by stimulating a motor nerve at one or more points along its course and recording the resulting compound muscle action potential (CMAP) with surface electrodes over the belly of the corresponding muscle. Each CMAP is a composite of all the muscle fiber action potentials of the nerve/muscle pair in question.

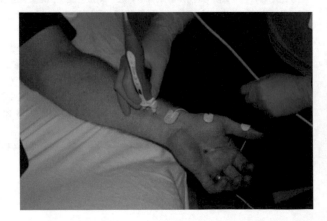

Fig. 8.1 Median motor nerve conduction study. Active recording electrode is over the abductor pollicis brevis muscle on the thenar eminence

Table 8.2 Parameters assessed during nerve conduction studies

Parameter	Unit	Measurement	Represents
Latency	ms	Distal latency: stimulus onset to initial response baseline deflection	Speed of fastest conduction fibers
		Peak latency: stimulus onset to midpoint of negative peak	Speed of slower conduction fibers
Amplitude	μV or mV	Baseline to negative peak	Number of muscle fibers or sensory fibers that depolarize
Conduction velocity	m/s	Calculated by dividing distance traveled by conduction time	Speed of fastest conduction fibers
Duration	ms	Initial baseline deflection to first baseline crossing (negative peak)	Synchronicity of muscle fiber depolarization

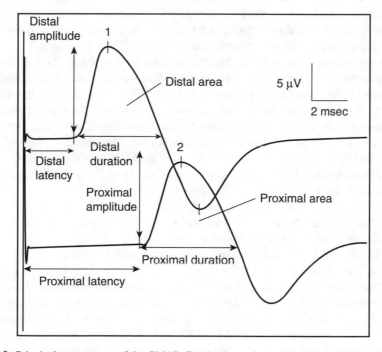

Fig. 8.2 Principal components of the CMAP. Conduction velocity is calculated by dividing distance traveled by conduction time (latency) between the onset of the proximal and distal responses

CMAP amplitude reflects the number of activated action potentials. A reduced CMAP amplitude indicates one of the following:

- Axon loss
- Distal conduction block
- Severe neuromuscular junction transmission failure
- Myofiber atrophy
- Submaximal nerve stimulation

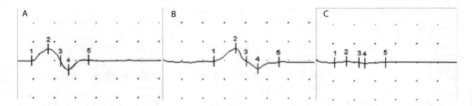

Fig. 8.3 (**a**) Normal motor conduction study (MCS) after distal stimulation; (**b**) MCS demonstrating prolonged latency due to demyelination; (**c**) MCS demonstrating reduced amplitude due to axon loss

While the CMAP itself does not indicate which of these is the reason, it can usually be inferred accurately from the findings of EMG, discussed below, and the clinical context. Because axonal neuropathy is far more common than the other pathologies listed, axon loss is the most common reason for low CMAP amplitude.

Latency reflects the speed of the fastest conducting nerve fibers (Fig. 8.3). Because latency measurements also include the time required for neuromuscular transmission and muscle fiber activation, latency measurements are not true assessments of velocity. For that reason, motor nerve conduction responses are typically obtained from at least two separate points along the nerve, and the motor nerve conduction velocity is then calculated using the distance between the points. Prolonged distal latency and slowed conduction velocity are findings that typically indicate demyelination, although mild slowing, typically >70% of the lower limit of normal, can also be seen with loss of the fastest-conducting axons [4].

Other important findings on motor NCS are *conduction block* and *temporal dispersion. Conduction block and temporal dispersion are findings that usually are indicative of an acquired demyelinating process.*

Conduction block is the failure of an action potential to conduct over a segment of nerve. Electrically this is demonstrated by showing a reduction in the recorded CMAP amplitude and area in a proximal stimulation site when compared to a distal stimulation site. While there is normally a small degree of amplitude attenuation with proximal stimulation, in most cases, pathologic conduction block is suspected when there is a reduction in proximal CMAP amplitude compared with distal CMAP amplitude by >30% and certainly when >50% in the absence of temporal dispersion, which is discussed below (Table 8.3) [5]. The degree of conduction block reflects the proportion of individual axons in which conduction is blocked.

Temporal dispersion refers to a pathologic increase in the duration of the CMAP. While normally the CMAP duration is modestly greater with proximal stimulation than distal stimulation, pathologic temporal dispersion reflects the fact that pathologic demyelination or remyelination can result in conduction velocity slowing without frank conduction block. When this occurs in all nerves to an equal degree, one would expect the CMAP duration to be unchanged but the conduction

Table 8.3 Electrophysiological criteria for conduction block

Conduction block	Definition
Definite[a]	Negative peak CMAP area reduction on proximal vs. distal stimulation of at least 50% whatever the nerve segment length (median, ulnar, and peroneal). Negative peak CMAP amplitude on stimulation of the distal part of the segment with motor CB must be >20% of the lower limit of normal and >1 mV and increase of proximal to distal negative peak CMAP duration must be ≤30%
Probable[a]	Negative peak CMAP area reduction of at least 30% over a long segment (e.g., wrist to elbow or elbow to axilla) of an upper limb nerve with increase of proximal to distal negative peak CMAP duration ≤30%
Probable[a]	Negative peak CMAP area reduction of at least 50% (same as definite) with an increase of proximal to distal negative peak CMAP duration >30%

Used with permission © John Wiley and Sons 2010 [5]
CMAP compound muscle action potential, *LLN* lower limit of normal
[a]Evidence for conduction block must be found at sites distinct from common entrapment or compression syndromes

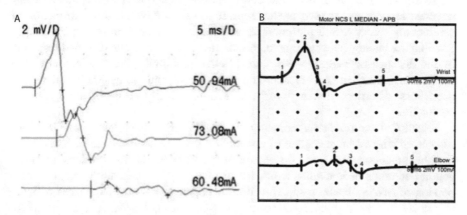

Fig. 8.4 Conduction block and temporal dispersion. (**a**) >50% amplitude decrement between the distalmost (top trace) and proximal (middle trace) stimuli, indicative of conduction block. In the most proximal (bottom trace) stimulus, marked temporal dispersion is noted. (**b**) Near-total conduction block and modest temporal dispersion are noted upon proximal stimulation (bottom trace)

velocity to be slowed. When this occurs in some axons more than others, the CMAP duration increases (pathologic temporal dispersion), because the range of conduction velocities, from some unaffected axons to others that are affected, broadens, and the components of the CMAP become desynchronized. If there is no associated conduction block, the area under the waveform remains essentially constant (Fig. 8.4).

Conduction block, temporal dispersion, and conduction velocity slowing that differ in severity between nerves and nerve segments are characteristic features of chronic inflammatory demyelinating polyneuropathy (CIDP). By contrast, in the demyelinating form of Charcot-Marie-Tooth (CMT1), conduction block and temporal dispersion are distinctly unusual, and the degree of conduction velocity slowing is typically uniform.

Sensory Nerve Conduction Studies

Sensory NCS are performed by depolarizing a nerve via electrical stimulation and recording the amplitude and latency of a resultant nerve action potential as it travels beneath an electrode at either a more proximal site along the nerve (*orthodromic* technique) or a more distal site (*antidromic* technique). The response recorded is known as the sensory nerve action potential (SNAP) [6].

There is no muscle or neuromuscular junction (NMJ) to navigate with sensory response recordings. As such, latency represents essentially the same information as conduction velocity, and the conduction velocity can be determined by simply dividing the latency between time of stimulation and onset of the recorded response by the distance between the two points. SNAP amplitudes are a reflection of the number of individual sensory fiber action potentials and are generally reduced in axon loss disorders. Latency (or conduction velocity) reflects the speed of conduction.

Recall that acquired demyelinating disorders (CIDP, its variants, and GBS) are associated with variable degrees of conduction slowing between axons, resulting in the phenomenon of temporal dispersion of the CMAP. Because the sensory nerve action potentials of individual axons are of relatively short duration, temporal dispersion of SNAPs leads to superposition of negative and positive phases of individual sensory axon potentials, resulting in *phase cancellation*. As a result, *while conduction velocity slowing, conduction block, and even temporal dispersion can be seen in sensory conduction studies, SNAP amplitudes are often reduced in acquired demyelinating disorders due to phase cancellation.* This is an important exception to the usual rule of thumb that axon loss results in low amplitudes, while myelin loss results in slow conduction.

Late Responses

Late responses (F waves and H reflexes) evaluate conduction along the entire course of the nerve, including the most proximal segments (Fig. 8.5) [7].

Fig. 8.5 Anatomy of late responses

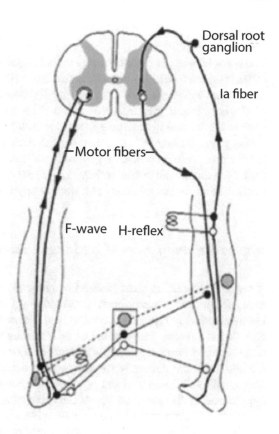

Dorsal root ganglion

Ia fiber

Motor fibers

F-wave   H-reflex

F Wave

Stimulation of a motor axon causes propagation of the response in an antidromic direction (i.e., impulse propagation in a direction opposite to normal physiology) to the anterior horn cell. When the action potential reaches the anterior horn cell, in a small proportion of cells, an orthodromic (i.e., impulse propagation in the normal physiologic direction) motor response traverses the initial segment after the refractory period and travels back to the recording electrode. Ten to 20 stimuli for recording F-wave responses are routinely performed from an individual nerve/muscle pair. Unlike the CMAP, F-wave configurations and latencies vary due to a polysynaptic response in the spinal cord, where Renshaw cells inhibit impulses from traveling the same path each time. F waves are generated with supramaximal stimulation and can be evaluated for minimum F-wave latency, persistence (number of recorded responses per group of stimuli), and chronodispersion (difference between the shortest and longest F-wave latencies). Prolonged minimum F-wave latency and increased chronodispersion generally indicate myelin injury. If F-wave latency is prolonged and distal nerve conduction velocity is normal, the presumption is that the myelin injury affects the proximal segment. Reduced persistence can be seen with axon injuries, loss of anterior horn cells, or proximal sites of conduction block.

H Reflex

The tibial H reflex is the electrophysiologic equivalent of the Achilles reflex. An H reflex is initiated with a submaximal stimulus to the tibial or, less commonly, median nerve. The response travels orthodromically along the Ia afferent fibers to the spinal cord where it activates motor efferents. The orthodromic motor response travels back to the recording electrode (soleus muscle). Unlike the F wave, H-reflex morphology and latency remain constant with each stimulus at a given intensity. Like the F wave, prolonged latency generally indicates myelin injury. Absent H reflexes have little diagnostic utility as they can be seen with axonal injuries, proximal conduction block, or occasionally as a normal physiologic phenomenon.

Interpretation of Nerve Conduction Study Parameters

Axon loss is typically characterized by reduced motor and sensory response amplitude with normal or near normal conduction velocity and distal latency (Table 8.4). Demyelination is typically characterized by prolonged distal latency and slowed conduction velocity with normal or near normal amplitude. Conduction block and temporal dispersion also usually reflect focal or segmental peripheral nerve demyelination and are generally indicative of a demyelinating process. As previously noted, both amplitude loss and conduction velocity slowing may be concomitantly appreciated in the same nerve. Widely available electrodiagnostic demyelinating criteria can be referenced when the pathophysiologic significance of mild or moderate degrees of conduction velocity slowing is uncertain (Table 8.5) [4].

Table 8.4 Interpretation of motor nerve conduction studies

Motor nerve abnormality	Alternative explanation
Findings suggesting axon loss	
Amplitude reduction	Submaximal stimulation
	Distal conduction block
	Severe neuromuscular junction transmission failure
	Myofiber atrophy
Findings suggesting demyelination	
Distal latency prolongation	Reduced limb temperature
Conduction velocity slowing	Loss of fastest conducting fibers
Conduction block	
Temporal dispersion	

Table 8.5 Electrodiagnostic criteria for CIDP according to 2010 EFNS/PNS criteria

(1) Definite: at least one of the following:
(a) Motor distal latency prolongation ≥50% above ULN in two nerves (excluding median neuropathy at the wrist)
(b) Reduction of motor conduction velocity ≥ 30% below LLN in two nerves
(c) Prolongation of F-wave latency ≥30% above ULN in two nerves (≥50% if amplitude of distal negative peak CMAP <80% of LLN values)
(d) Absence of F waves in two nerves if these nerves have distal negative peak CMAP amplitudes ≥20% of LLN + ≥1 other demyelinating parameter[a] in ≥1 other nerve
(e) Partial motor conduction block[b]: ≥50% amplitude reduction of the proximal negative peak CMAP relative to distal, if distal negative peak CMAP ≥20% of LLN, in two nerves, or in one nerve + ≥1 other demyelinating parameter[a] in ≥1 other nerve
(f) Abnormal temporal dispersion (>30% duration increase between the proximal and distal negative peak CMAP) in ≥2 nerves
(g) Distal CMAP duration (interval between onset of the first negative peak and return to baseline of the last negative peak) increase in ≥1 nerve (median ≥ 6.6 ms, ulnar ≥6.7 ms, peroneal ≥7.6 ms, tibial ≥8.8 ms) + ≥1 other demyelinating parameter[a] in ≥1 other nerve
(2) Probable
Partial motor conduction block[b]: ≥30% amplitude reduction of the proximal negative peak CMAP relative to distal, excluding the posterior tibial nerve, if distal negative peak CMAP ≥20% of LLN, in two nerves, or in one nerve + ≥1 other demyelinating parameter[a] in ≥1 other nerve
(3) Possible
As in (1) but in only one nerve

Used with permission © John Wiley and Sons 2010 [4]
To apply criteria, median, ulnar, peroneal (stimulated below the fibular head), and tibial nerves on one side are tested. If criteria are not fulfilled, the same nerves are tested at the other side, and/or ulnar and median nerves are stimulated at the axilla and Erb's point. Temperatures are maintained to ≥33 °C palm and ≥30 °C external malleolus
[a]Any nerve meeting of any of the criteria (a–g)
[b]Conduction block is not considered in the ulnar nerve across the elbow and at least 50% amplitude reduction between Erb's point and the wrist is required for probable conduction block

Localization Using Nerve Conduction Studies

Nerve conduction studies are a collection of data from individual nerves. Hence, using NCS to localize or characterize pathology requires obtaining sufficient data to answer the referring provider's diagnostic question.

- If the question relates to a possible polyneuropathy, a sufficient number of nerve conduction studies from both sides and upper and lower limbs are needed to determine whether the problem is length dependent, non-length dependent, or multifocal.
- If the question relates to a possible single lesion of peripheral nerve, plexus, or root, nerve conduction studies referable to the structure in question are needed. If they are abnormal, nerve conduction studies of neighboring or contralateral structures determine whether the findings reflect a single lesion or a polyneuropathy.

- If NCS are abnormal, it is imperative to determine whether the findings are motor only, sensory only, or both.
- If NCS are abnormal, it is imperative to determine whether the primary process is axon loss or a disorder of myelin, using the principles discussed above.

In this way, NCS supplement the neurologic examination in establishing the distribution, modalities affected, and primary pathology in neurogenic disorders. Note that motor NCS can also be abnormal in disorders of muscle and neuromuscular transmission, diagnoses that become clear with EMG, RNS, and the clinical context.

Localization of pathology based on nerve conduction studies requires detailed knowledge of peripheral nervous system anatomy, including the course of individual named nerves through their corresponding plexus and nerve roots. Lesion localization based on nerve conduction studies is performed by recognizing NCS abnormalities with intersecting anatomical localizations as well as identification of focal abnormalities across discrete nerve segments. Detection of focal slowing or conduction block across a short segment of nerve indicates pathology at that site.

Sensory Symptoms with Normal Sensory Conduction Studies

The motor nerve cell body is within the spinal cord at the anterior horn cell, but the sensory cell bodies are in the peripheral nervous system at the dorsal root ganglion (DRG). As such, peripheral lesions proximal to the dorsal root ganglion may cause sensory symptoms in the corresponding area but will leave the peripheral nerve components structurally intact. *Hence, normal sensory nerve conduction studies in people with large-fiber-type sensory loss should alert the clinician to preganglionic localization. For example, patients with sensory symptoms due to radiculopathy have normal SNAP amplitudes, while patients with sensory symptoms due to axonal neuropathy typically have reduced SNAP amplitudes. Recall also that sensory NCS only evaluate large myelinated axons. Sensory NCS are, by definition, normal in small fiber neuropathy.*

Electromyography

Needle electromyography (EMG) refers to the recording of electrical activity of skeletal muscle using an intramuscular needle recording electrode [2]. The electrical characteristics of the muscle at rest and during activity can be interpreted by the electrodiagnostic physician. The muscles studied with EMG will vary depending upon the initial diagnostic query and the coalescence of information obtained by the physician during the electrodiagnostic test. *With each muscle sampled, spontaneous activity, motor unit potential morphology, and motor unit potential recruitment should be analyzed* (Table 8.6) [8].

Table 8.6 Parameters assessed during needle EMG

Parameter	Muscle activity	Observation
Spontaneous activity	Rest	Presence or absence of spontaneous discharges
MUAP morphology	Low-level activation	Size, duration, and complexity of the MUAPs
Recruitment	Mid- or high-level activation	Firing pattern and rate of MUAPs

EMG Procedures

After the skin is cleaned with an antiseptic solution (usually alcohol), a small disposable concentric needle electrode is inserted into the muscle. The electrode consists of a fine wire, which serves as the active electrode, surrounded by a cannula, which serves as the reference electrode. Unlike NCS, which record either nerve or compound muscle action potentials but are used principally as a test of nerve function, EMG directly records only the electrical potentials generated by depolarization of muscle cells. The electromyographer first assesses *spontaneous activity*, which represents muscle cell discharges at rest, and then assesses *volitional activity, or the configuration and firing patterns of individual motor unit action potentials (MUAPs)*, which represent the near-simultaneous discharge of all muscle cells innervated by a single axon, and hence reflect the structure and function of a motor unit.

Note that the EMG electrode only registers electrical activity from a small surrounding area; hence, although the electromyographer does sample several areas by repositioning the needle, needle electromyography is subject to sampling error and can easily miss abnormalities if they are nonuniform and in a large muscle. Furthermore, some components of a motor unit may extend beyond the recording area of the electrode.

The electrical activity is amplified and transduced into both visual and auditory signals, so the examiner can both hear and see the electromyographic findings.

- *Spontaneous activity is assessed first* by moving the needle through the muscle with small quick movements. Multiple locations of the muscle should be sampled with a single-needle insertion. At each sampling site, the examiner pauses for several seconds and notes any abnormalities. Types of spontaneous activity are outlined below and in Table 8.7.
- *Motor unit action potentials (MUAP) are evaluated next.* With the needle in a fixed position, the patient minimally contracts the muscle until an action potential of a single motor unit is observed. Each MUAP is assessed for amplitude (peak to peak, mV), duration (ms), and number of phases (turns or baseline crossings). Multiple individual MUAPs should be analyzed.
- *Recruitment is assessed next* by asking the patient to increase the level of contraction (Fig. 8.6). The number and speed with which additional MUAPs appear define recruitment.

Table 8.7 Spontaneous activity during needle EMG

	Amplitude	Duration	Morphology	Rhythm	Sound	Interpretation
End plate noise	10–20 μV	0.5–1 ms	Simple	Irregular	Seashell	Normal
End plate spikes	100–300 μV	2–4 ms	Simple	Irregular	Popcorn	Normal
Fibrillation potentials and PSW	10–100 μV	1–5 ms	Simple	Regular at 1–50 Hz	Rain on a tin roof	Spontaneous muscle fiber contraction
Fasciculation	Often ≥200 μV	Often ≥10 ms	Simple or complex	Irregular at 0.1 to 10 Hz	Pop	Spontaneous single motor unit discharge
CRD	100 μV–1 mV	Variable	Complex	Regular at 20–150 Hz	Machine like	Ephaptic transmission between adjacent fibers
Myotonia	Waxing and waning	Waxing and waning	Simple	Irregular 20–150 Hz	Dive bomber	Muscle membrane instability
Myokymia	Variable	Variable	Simple or complex	Regular or irregular 5–60 Hz	March	Spontaneous or ephaptic motor nerve discharge
Neuromyotonia	Waning	Variable	Simple or complex	Irregular 150–250 Hz	Ping	Motor axon hyperexcitability

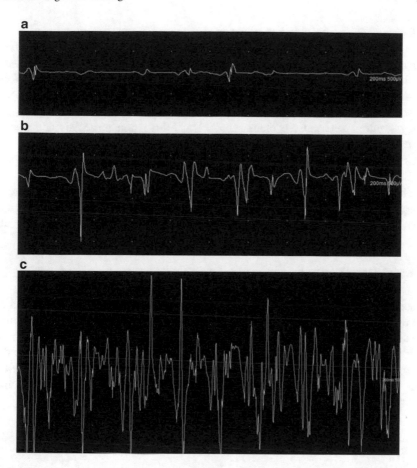

Fig. 8.6 Normal motor unit activation patterns at minimal (**a**), moderate (**b**), and full activation (**c**)

Spontaneous Activity

The term "spontaneous activity" applies to electromyographic discharges that can be recorded with the muscle at rest and is distinguished from recordings made from voluntarily activated motor units. Most are abnormal and have specific etiologic implications. By far the most common are fibrillation potentials and positive sharp waves. The following are the types of spontaneous activity.

Fibrillation Potentials and Positive Sharp Waves

Fibrillation potentials and positive sharp waves are action potentials of a single muscle fiber undergoing spontaneous depolarization. Although they have different names and appearances, their pathologic significance is essentially indistinguishable. As noted they are by far the most common type of abnormal spontaneous activity. Fibrillation potentials and positive sharp waves *indicate either denervation, as occurs in axon loss, or loss of the integrity of muscle membrane, as occurs in many myopathies, such as muscular dystrophy or rhabdomyolysis.* By contrast they are not seen in neuropathies and myopathies with preserved neuromuscular junctions and muscle cell membranes, such as pure demyelination and muscle channelopathies. Fibrillation potentials and positive sharp waves do not develop until 2–3 weeks after axonal injury, so in the acute phase, it can be difficult to distinguish axon loss from conduction block on the basis of EMG alone.

Fibrillation potentials and positive sharp waves are scored as follows: 0 (none), 1+ (single train of potentials longer than 2 s in 2 areas), 2+ (moderate numbers in 3 or more areas), 3+ (many potentials in all areas), and 4+ (full interference pattern of potentials).

Fasciculation Potentials

Fasciculation potentials reflect a spontaneous discharge of a single motor axon and are the electrophysiologic signature of a clinical fasciculation. Because they reflect the simultaneous contraction of all muscle fibers innervated by a single axon, they are much larger than fibrillation potentials, which represent the contraction of only a single muscle cell. They often sound like a large "pop." Fasciculation potentials may be benign but also occur in disorders of axonal excitability, polyneuropathies, and anterior horn cell disorders.

Complex Repetitive Discharges (CRD)

CRDs are stereotyped, recurrent discharges of several adjoining muscle fibers. They have a constant frequency and a very distinct sound reminiscent of mechanical equipment. CRDs probably arise from ephaptic transmission between adjacent denervated fibers. CRDs are most commonly seen in chronic neurogenic disorders in which there has been denervation, reinnervation, and subsequent denervation.

Myotonic Discharges

Myotonic discharges are high-frequency trains of fibrillation-like potentials that vary in frequency and amplitude in a waxing and waning patterns. These regular variations result in a characteristic sound often likened to that of a "dive bomber," or the Doppler effect superimposed on the sound of a rapidly firing airplane engine. Myotonic discharges occur with disorders in muscle fiber membrane channels, including myotonic dystrophy and non-dystrophic channelopathies such as myotonia congenital and paramyotonia congenita.

Neuromyotonia

Neuromyotonia arises from hyperexcitability of a single peripheral motor axon. It is characterized by a very high-frequency discharge (100–300 Hz, faster than myotonic discharges) of a motor unit, partial motor unit, or single-fiber potentials. Clinical syndromes associated with electrical neuromyotonia include autoimmune Isaac's syndrome due to voltage-gated potassium channel antibodies.

Myokymia

Myokymia is a spontaneous, rhythmic, regular, or irregular discharge of groups of motor units that produce the clinical appearance of quivering in the muscles (grouped fasciculations). The discharges fire repetitively in single or grouped units at a uniform rate. They often sound like a group of soldiers marching. Myokymia can occur with chronic disorders of peripheral nerve and is most commonly seen in radiation nerve injury.

End Plate Noise and Spikes

End plate noise and spikes are normal spontaneous activity. The activity can be heard when the needle electrode is close to end plates. End plate noise has a characteristic "seashell" sound, whereas end plate spikes are irregular and sometimes sound like "popcorn." These reflect release of subthreshold quantities of acetylcholine across the neuromuscular junction and are the only type of spontaneous activity that is always normal.

Motor Unit Action Potential Morphology

Normal Motor Unit Action Potentials

MUAPs have a characteristic appearance. MUAP duration is defined as the time from initial deflection from baseline to the final return to baseline and is normally between 5 and 15 ms. Duration reflects the number of muscle fibers within a motor unit and the dispersion of fiber depolarizations over time. Short or brief duration MUAPs are classically seen in myopathic disorders, reflecting the presence of fewer functional muscle cells. Duration typically lengthens with increasing numbers of muscle fibers in a motor unit, such as when neurogenic reinnervation follows denervation. Duration lengthening can also be seen with increasing age and with decreased temperature. Audibly, duration is associated with pitch. Short duration MUAPs sound crisp and high pitched, like a sound from a small drum, while long-duration MUAPs sound dull and low-pitched, like a sound from a bass drum.

MUAP amplitude is generally between 200 μV to 2 mV, measured peak to peak, although it can vary depending on the muscle sampled. Amplitude represents only those few fibers closest to the needle, rather than the total number of fibers, and reflects muscle fiber density or muscle fiber diameter. That said, MUAP amplitude and duration are highly correlated, and both are increased most commonly due to increased motor unit size due to reinnervation. Increased MUAP amplitude can also be appreciated in chronic myopathies with muscle fiber hypertrophy. Audibly, amplitude is associated with volume. Larger amplitude MUAPs sound louder.

Polyphasia is a measure of muscle fiber firing synchronicity. MUAPs generally have ≤5 phases (baseline crossings). MUAPs from muscle fibers with poor synchronicity (muscle fibers firing at different times) have increased phases and turns (direction changes). This can occur with both neurogenic and myopathic disorders. Some degree of polyphasia is seen in normal muscle. Pathologic increased polyphasia requires at least 10% of the sampled muscle fibers to have >5 phases.

Abnormal Motor Unit Action Potentials

Changes in motor unit potential morphology can give clues to the underlying mechanism of injury and the duration of injury (Table 8.8). Generally speaking, high-amplitude, long-duration motor unit potentials with or without increased polyphasia develop after denervation and reinnervation (Fig. 8.7a). As part of the reinnervation process, collateral sprouting extends axons to denervated muscle fibers, effectively increasing the number of muscle fibers of that motor unit. More muscle fibers within a given motor unit lead to larger MUAPs with longer durations and increased polyphasia. In primary muscle disease, individual muscle fibers are injured, resulting in a reduced number of muscle fibers within any given motor unit. With fewer muscle fibers to contribute to the compound action potential, amplitudes become small and durations short (Fig. 8.7b). Polyphasia may increase as well. Rarely, chronic myopathies with muscle fiber hypertrophy can have a mixed appearance with both large and small MUAPs.

Motor Unit Recruitment

Recruitment refers to the successive activation of motor units with increasing strength of voluntary muscle contraction [9]. With minimal muscle activation, a single motor unit becomes activated with a firing rate of about 5 Hz. With increased voluntary effort (central drive), the single motor unit fires faster to increase force generation. When the firing rate increases to about 10 Hz, another motor unit is activated or *recruited*. As central drive increases further, the first MUAP increases firing to 15 Hz, the second to 10 Hz, and then another MUAP is recruited. This pattern

Table 8.8 Motor unit action potential morphology

Parameter	Represents	Normal	Pathologic increase when	Pathologic decrease when
Duration[a]	Number of muscle fibers in motor unit	5–15 ms	Neurogenic reinnervation after denervation	Myopathy
Amplitude[a]	Muscle fiber density or muscle fiber size	100 μV–2 mV	Neurogenic reinnervation; muscle fiber hypertrophy	Myopathy without muscle fiber hypertrophy
Polyphasia[a]	Synchronicity of muscle fiber firing	<5 phases	Early neurogenic reinnervation; chronic reinnervation; acute or chronic myopathy	No pathologic significance

[a]Additional variations may be seen depending on muscle selected, age, and temperature

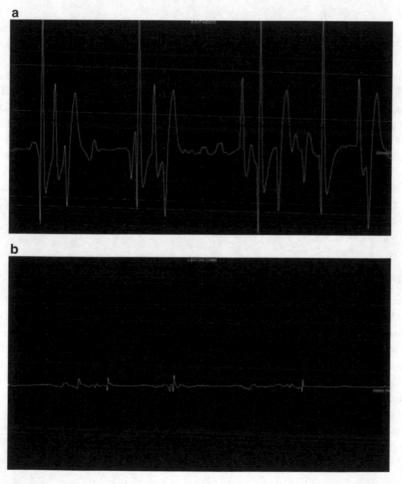

Fig. 8.7 (**a**) High-amplitude, long-duration, "neurogenic" motor unit potentials reflecting reinnervation; (**b**) low-amplitude, short-duration "myopathic" motor unit potentials

of recruitment is continued until MUAPs reach tetanic frequency of about 30–50 Hz, with the ratio of firing frequency to the number of different MUAPs firing remaining at approximately 5:1.

Neurogenic injuries (axon loss or conduction block) result in *reduced recruitment*. Reduced recruitment means that the firing rate of individual motor units is normal, but as central drive increases, there is failure to add more motor units. The result is that the electromyographer sees and hears only a few MUAPs that fire rapidly.

Myogenic injuries typically result in *early recruitment*. When there is a loss of individual muscle fibers, the motor unit generates less force. The motor units remain intact and so to increase power motor units must fire earlier than would be expected with a normal 5:1 recruitment ratio. Early recruitment means that the number of MUAPs firing is increased for the degree of force generated.

Interpreting Electrodiagnostic Findings

As indicated above, NCS identify the distribution, modalities affected, and pathophysiology of neurogenic disorders and will often demonstrate reduced CMAPs in myopathic disorders. EMG will usually reliably distinguish myopathic, acute neurogenic, and chronic neurogenic processes based upon the features of spontaneous activity and the configuration and firing pattern of voluntarily active MUAPs. When investigating a focal lesion such as a mononeuropathy or radiculopathy, the electromyographer will study several muscles that share root or nerve innervation and make an anatomic diagnosis based upon the common innervation pattern of affected muscles. The electromyographic features of common neuromuscular conditions are outlined in Table 8.9.

Summary

The key to a successful NCS/EMG study begins with understanding what question is being explored. The electrodiagnostic clinician can then plan a well-organized study that evolves with the findings as they emerge. Many abnormalities might be uncovered during an NCS/EMG study. An understanding of these abnormalities provides the clinician with an important foundation to determine localization, pathophysiology, severity, and chronicity.

Table 8.9 Interpreting electrodiagnostic findings

	Nerve conduction studies		Electromyography			
	CMAP amplitude	SNAP amplitude	Spontaneous activity (Fibs/PSW)	MUAP morphology	Recruitment	Comment
Hyperacute axon loss (<1 week)	Normal	Normal	Absent	Normal	Reduced	Before Wallerian degeneration
Acute axon loss (days–weeks)	Decreased	Decreased[a]	Absent	Normal	Reduced	Wallerian degeneration occurred, but fibs may take 2–6 weeks
Subacute axon (weeks–2 months)	Decreased	Decreased[a]	Present	Normal	Reduced	Denervation potentials present
Chronic axon loss with reinnervation (>2 months)	Decreased	Decreased[a]	Absent	Large, long	Reduced	MUAP remodeling
Myopathic	Normal or decreased	Normal	Increased or normal	Small, brief	Early	Variable depending on type and duration

[a]If postganglionic

Fibs fibrillation potentials, *MUAP* motor action unit potential, *PSW* positive sharp waves

References

1. Barboi AC, Barkhaus PE. Electrodiagnostic testing in neuromuscular disorders. Neurol Clin. 2004;22(3):619–41.
2. https://www.aanem.org/getmedia/65934187-d91e-4336-9f3c-50522449e565/Model-Policy.pdf.
3. Gutmann L. Pearls and pitfalls in the use of electromyography and nerve conduction studies. Semin Neurol. 2003;23(1):77–82.
4. Van den Bergh PY, Hadden RD, Bouche P, et al. European Federation of Neurological Societies/Peripheral Nerve Society guideline on management of chronic inflammatory demyelinating polyradiculoneuropathy: report of a joint task force of the European Federation of Neurological Societies and the Peripheral Nerve Society – first revision. Eur J Neurol. 2010;17(3):356–63.
5. Joint Task Force of the EFNS and the PNS. European Federation of Neurologic Societies/Peripheral Nerve Society guideline on management of multifocal motor neuropathy. Report of a joint task force of the European Federation of Neurological Societies and the Peripheral Nerve Society--first revision. J Peripher Nerv Syst. 2010;15(4):295–301.
6. Wilbourn AJ. Sensory nerve conduction studies. J Clin Neurophysiol. 1994;11(6):584–601.
7. Fisher MA. H reflexes and F waves. Fundamentals, normal and abnormal patterns. Neurol Clin. 2002;20(2):339–60.
8. Daube JR, Rubin DI. Needle electromyography. Muscle Nerve. 2009;39(2):244–70.
9. Enoka RM. Morphological features and activation patterns of motor units. J Clin Neurophysiol. 1995;12(6):538–59.

Chapter 9
Ventilatory Management in Neuromuscular Disease

Deanna Diebold

Abbreviations

FVC   Forced vital capacity
MEP   Maximal expiratory pressure
MIP   Maximal inspiratory pressure
NIV   Non-invasive ventilation

Key Points
- Rapidly progressive neuromuscular conditions such as Guillain-Barre syndrome and myasthenia gravis often require ICU monitoring.
- More slowly progressive conditions can usually be managed in the outpatient setting, but patients eventually require ventilatory support.
- Respiratory infections can be life-threatening in these patients and may require early and aggressive treatment.
- Airway clearance therapy is an important adjunct in the treatment of respiratory infections.
- Both quality of life and survival can be improved with optimal management of hypoventilation and respiratory infections.

In patients with neuromuscular disease, respiratory complications are a major source of morbidity and mortality. These complications stem from weakness of inspiratory and expiratory muscles as well as dysfunction of bulbar musculature, leading to hypoventilation, weak cough, and inadequate airway protection. Optimal management of respiratory function in these patients improves both quality of life and survival [1–4].

The advent of new modalities for treatment of chronic respiratory failure, such as noninvasive ventilation (NIV/BiPAP®), has revolutionized the management of neuromuscular respiratory failure. Whereas therapeutic nihilism once was the

D. Diebold, MD (✉)
University of Minnesota, Pulmonary, Critical Care, and Sleep Medicine,
Minneapolis, MN, USA
e-mail: deibo001@umn.edu

© Springer International Publishing AG, part of Springer Nature 2018   183
D. Walk (ed.), *Clinical Handbook of Neuromuscular Medicine*,
https://doi.org/10.1007/978-3-319-67116-1_9

dominant paradigm, the current standard of care includes much more proactive monitoring and treatment of respiratory complications, resulting in significant benefit to patients.

Note that *respiration* is a cellular event, while *ventilation* refers to the mechanical act of gas exchange in the lung. Hence, this chapter is, strictly speaking, about ventilatory function and management. However, the medical literature uses the term "respiratory" so widely in this context that in this chapter we will use these terms interchangeably.

Acute Respiratory Failure: Rapidly Progressive Neuromuscular Conditions

Guillain-Barre syndrome (GBS) is classically associated with rapid progression, and in a certain percentage of patients, this leads to frank respiratory failure necessitating intubation and mechanical ventilation. Exacerbations of myasthenia gravis can also present with respiratory failure. Less often, respiratory failure is the presenting symptom of a more slowly progressive neuromuscular process.

Patients with rapidly progressive conditions or frank respiratory failure can sometimes be managed using NIV, but they often require intubation. Because of this, they require close monitoring in an intensive care unit. Monitor bedside respiratory parameters as frequently as every 4 hours in severe cases, and consider ventilatory support if:

- *Vital capacity < 20 cc/kg ideal body weight*
- *Maximal inspiratory pressure (MIP) < 30*
- *Maximal expiratory pressure (MEP) < 40*

The 20/30/40 rule [5] (above), along with trajectory of illness and clinical judgement, is sometimes used to help guide the clinician in determining whether a patient requires ventilatory support. Other more complex scoring systems have been developed but have not been shown to be superior [6]. *Any patient with altered mental status resulting in inability to protect the airway requires endotracheal intubation.*

Acute Respiratory Failure: Non-neuromuscular Exacerbation

Patients with underlying neuromuscular weakness from any cause are more susceptible to respiratory failure with superimposed illness. The most common respiratory illness in these patients is viral or bacterial infection, but heart failure and other causes are also seen. Especially in the case of infection, *airway clearance therapy* is crucial in addition to aggressive supportive care and antibiotics. Several modalities are available for airway clearance:

- Manually assisted cough, known colloquially as "quad cough," is a properly timed abdominal thrust maneuver that can be performed by a respiratory therapist (RT) or caregiver. Similar to the Heimlich maneuver used for choking victims, this increases expiratory force in order to expel mucus.
- Lung volume recruitment, also known as "breath stacking," requires intact glottis function and can be done with manual assistance with a bag valve mask or by the patient taking a series of breaths without exhaling between each breath.
- Insufflator-exsufflator or "cough assist" is a machine that delivers a positive pressure breath through a mask or mouthpiece that is held over the nose and mouth of the patient. After this large inhalation is delivered, there is a pause followed by negative flow from the machine, thereby moving mucus upward from the lower airways. The use of this device is sometimes supplemented by a manually assisted cough.
- High-frequency chest wall oscillation (HFCWO) can be done using a hand-held vibratory device or through the use of a VEST®. In patients with neuromuscular disease, it is recommended that one of the above modalities be paired with HFCWO to expel the mucus once it has been mobilized.
- EzPAP® and MetaNeb® are examples of newer devices that can be used to help with airway clearance. EzPAP® provides positive airway pressure without the exsufflation of the cough assist machine. MetaNeb® provides oscillatory airflow within the airways. Both can be used in conjunction with inhaled bronchodilators or mucolytics. *Mucomyst®* or inhaled N-acetylcysteine (NAC) is the most commonly used mucolytic, and it is sometimes helpful in patients with thick secretions. One potential side effect of NAC is bronchospasm, so it must be used with caution. Thick secretions can also be helped with improved hydration of the patient.

Tracheostomy is indicated in patients who have failed noninvasive modalities of airway clearance. This allows for deep suctioning of secretions during times of increased mucus production, and it can also facilitate mechanical ventilation if a cuffed tracheostomy tube is used. Patients can do well for many years with tracheostomy, although the presence of the tracheostomy tube puts them at risk for airway infection. It is also more difficult to swallow with a tracheostomy tube present, so in certain cases, tracheostomy will raise the risk of aspiration.

Chronic Respiratory Failure

Patients with more slowly progressive neuromuscular diseases such as ALS, DMD, and SMA are usually cared for in the outpatient setting. ALS manifests a very variable phenotype, with respiratory failure early or late in a patient's course depending largely upon the point at which the condition spreads to the cervical and thoracic motor neuron pools (Fig. 9.1). Patients with DMD progress in a somewhat more predictable fashion, and respiratory failure becomes a concern once they are nonambulatory. In SMA II, diaphragm function is often relatively spared, so respiratory failure develops later.

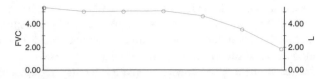

Fig. 9.1 Representative change in FVC over time in a person with ALS. Each point represents a successive 3-month interval. Ventilatory function in ALS, like bulbar and limb function, is normal until the disease processes reach the relevant motor neuron pools and then progress in a roughly predictable fashion

In the absence of coexisting cardiopulmonary disease, hypercarbia (PaCO2 > 50 mmHg) precedes hypoxemia (PaO2 < 60 mmHg). Therefore, hypoxemia in the absence of hypercarbia should prompt separate evaluation for cardiac or pulmonary abnormalities. Monitoring oxygen saturation alone is inadequate in the evaluation of patients with neuromuscular disease, as hypoxemia is a late finding. *Supplemental O2 without NIV in these patients is usually contraindicated and should be used with extreme caution.*

Hypercarbia in neuromuscular disease first occurs during REM sleep. This is due to the normal processes of rapid eye movement (REM) hypotonia (of all muscles excluding the diaphragm), along with reduced sensitivity of CO2 chemoreceptors. As muscle weakness progresses, hypoventilation is found during non-REM sleep and finally during wakefulness. *The symptoms of hypoventilation are insidious and can often go unrecognized by patients.* They include:

- *Frequent nocturnal awakenings*, usually without perceived dyspnea, often manifesting as nocturia or just generally "restless" sleep
- *Nonrestorative sleep* or longer sleep requirement than "normal" for that patient
- *Morning confusion and/or headaches*
- *Orthopnea*, often not mentioned, even if the patient has been progressively raising the head of his/her bed or even sleeping in a recliner
- *Daytime dyspnea, which* is a relatively rare early finding in patients with neuromuscular disease

Pulmonary function testing in patients with neuromuscular disease will typically reveal a restrictive pattern – symmetric reduction in FEV1 and FVC, with FEV1/FVC ratio > 0.7. Supine FVC is a more sensitive marker than upright FVC. In patients with significant diaphragm dysfunction, there is typically a 20% or greater reduction in supine vs upright FVC. MIP and MEP are also commonly used, and a MIP value of −60 or worse is associated with nocturnal hypoventilation. Reduced MEP and peak cough flow (PCF) are associated with reduced cough effectiveness. If full PFTs are performed, reduced ERV and elevated RV may be seen. A normal DLCO would be expected (if patient is able to adequately perform the maneuver), and reduction in DLCO (<70% predicted) should prompt consideration of evaluation for intrinsic cardiopulmonary disease. Principal PFT parameters in neuromuscular disease are listed in Table 9.1, and representative studies are in Fig. 9.2.

--- SPIROMETRY ---	Actual	Pred	%Pred	--- SPIROMETRY ---	Actual	Pred	%Pred
FVC (L)	*2.68	4.25	*63	FVC (L)	*1.84	5.54	*33
FEVI (L)	*2.35	3.27	*71	FEVI (L)	*1.72	4.28	*40
FEVI /FVC (%)	87		77	FEVI /FVC (%)	*93		78
FEF Max (L/sec)	6.62	8.55	77	FEF Max (L/sec)	*2.55	10.52	*24
FEF 25-75% (L/sec)	3.45	2.65	130	FEF 25-75% (L/sec)	2.17	3.65	59
FIVC (L)	2.66			FIVC (L)	1.45		
FIF Max (L/sec)	4.49	7.04	63	FIF Max (L/sec)	*2.69	8.44	*31
FIVC (L)	2.66			FIVC (L)	1.45		
Expiratory Time (sec)	7.84			Expiratory Time (sec)	1.78		
--- LUNG MECHANICS ---				--- LUNG MECHANICS ---			
MEP (cmH20)	90			MEP (cmH20)	25		
MIP (cmH20)	-65			MIP (cmH20)	-40		

Fig. 9.2 PFTs in people with neuromuscular disease. Note reduced FVC without reduction in FEV1/FVC. MEP and MIP are normal in the patient on the left, who has only moderate reduction in FVC of 63% of predicted, and abnormal in the patient on the right, whose FVC is markedly reduced at 33% of predicted

Table 9.1 Principal pulmonary function parameters in neuromuscular disease

Parameter	Clinical implication in neuromuscular disease
FVC	Ventilatory muscle weakness
Supine FVC	Diaphragmatic weakness; increased likelihood of orthopnea and nocturnal hypoventilation
MIP	Increased likelihood of orthopnea and nocturnal hypoventilation; on occasion becomes abnormal when FVC still normal
MEP	Reduced cough effectiveness
PCF	Reduced cough effectiveness

Polysomnography (PSG) is a valuable tool for diagnosing nocturnal hypoventilation. This should be done in a sleep lab that has experience with transcutaneous CO2 monitoring and NIV/BiPAP® titration. *Overnight oximetry* can also be helpful; oxygen desaturations lasting at least 1 minute could be consistent with hypoventilation.

Treatment of patients with chronic neuromuscular respiratory failure is largely supportive, and current treatment modalities are quite effective. Nocturnal NIV is usually started based on a combination of symptoms (which can be quite subtle, as noted above) and abnormalities in pulmonary function, PSG, or overnight oximetry. In the United States, insurance generally covers NIV in patients with neuromuscular disease who demonstrate one of the following:

- FVC < 50% predicted.
- MIP < 60 cm H2O.
- Daytime PaCO2 > 45 mmHg.
- Overnight oximetry shows desaturation <88% for ≥5 minutes.

If none of these conditions is met but nocturnal hypoventilation is still suspected, a PSG should be considered.

Continuous positive airway pressure (CPAP) should not be used in patients with significant neuromuscular weakness. CPAP can be continued in patients with preserved respiratory muscle strength and pre-existing obstructive sleep apnea; however this should be closely monitored and transition to NIV made as respiratory muscle strength deteriorates.

Invasive Mechanical Ventilation

Continuous mechanical ventilation, usually with tracheostomy, is an option for people with ventilatory failure due to neuromuscular disease. If bulbar function permits, speech and even swallowing can continue in some circumstances. Invasive mechanical ventilation in the setting of ventilatory failure does however increase the complexity and cost of care. When ventilatory failure from neuromuscular disease can be anticipated, people living with neuromuscular disease need to consider numerous factors, including their quality of life, goals of care, neuromuscular prognosis, availability of caregivers, personal and family circumstances, and resources, before making a decision. A full discussion of this issue is beyond the scope of this chapter.

As in acutely ill hospitalized patients, airway clearance therapy needs to be considered in the outpatient setting. Some patients without chronic chest congestion benefit from regular use of airway clearance modalities, but all patients should at least be aware of the need for assisted airway clearance during times of illness to prevent complications, including hospitalization and death.

Supportive Care and General Health Measures for People with Chronic Ventilatory Failure

Prevention of acute illness is also important to discuss in the outpatient setting – this includes:

- Smoking cessation.
- Yearly influenza vaccination.
- Pneumococcal vaccination – current CDC recommendations are one dose for patients with risk factors and a repeat dose at age 65 if >5 years have elapsed since the first dose.
- Avoidance of ill contacts.
- Early antimicrobial therapy – somewhat controversial.

Perioperative Management

Patients with neuromuscular weakness are at increased risk for respiratory complications with surgical procedures, due to potentiation of respiratory muscle weakness in the setting of sedation or anesthesia. Nonessential procedures should be avoided due to this increased risk. The use of NIV in the perioperative period can mitigate the risk of anesthetic-related respiratory suppression when surgical procedures are necessary, however.

Patients who tolerate NIV at baseline will have an improved risk profile compared with those who do not tolerate NIV. The patient should bring his/her home NIV machine and mask interface to the hospital or surgery center. If the patient will be intubated for the procedure, he or she can be extubated directly to NIV in the postoperative area and continue on NIV until fully recovered from anesthesia. If the patient will not be intubated for the procedure, NIV can be used continuously during the procedure and throughout the recovery period.

Certain procedures (such as endoscopic gastrostomy tube placement) require a patient to lie supine without full facemask NIV during the procedure. This can significantly complicate the timing of these procedures and even make them impossible at later stages of the disease, unless the patient also wishes to undergo tracheostomy. Therefore, the discussion of gastrostomy, especially in patients with ALS who will likely develop dysphagia during the course of their illness, should happen while ventilatory function is still relatively preserved.

Conclusions

Respiratory complications are common in neuromuscular conditions, and they cause significant morbidity and mortality in these patients. However, effective therapies are available and can lead to improved quality and duration of life when used properly.

References

1. Ambrosino N, et al. Chronic respiratory care for neuromuscular diseases in adults. Eur Respir J. 2009;34.444–57.
2. Miller RG, et al. Practice parameter update in ALS. Neurology. 2009;73:1218–26. Bach JR, et al. Extubation of patients with neuromuscular weakness. Chest. 2010;137:1033–9.
3. Benditt JO, Boitano LJ. Pulmonary issues in patients with chronic neuromuscular disease. Am J Respir Crit Care Med. 2013;187(10):1046–55.
4. Oana S, Mukherji J. Acute and chronic respiratory failure. In: Handbook of clinical neurology. Vol. 119, 3rd series, chapter 19; 2014.
5. Lawn ND, Fletcher DD, Henderson RD, Wolter TD, Widjicks EF. Anticipating mechanical ventilation in Guillain-Barre syndrome. Arch Neurol. 2001;58:893–8.
6. Kannan Kanikannan MA, Durga P, Venigalla NK, Kandadai RM, Jabeen SA, Borgohain R. Simple bedside predictors of mechanical ventilation in patients with Guillain-Barre syndrome. J Crit Care. 2014;29:219–23.

Chapter 10
Genetic Testing in Neuromuscular Disease

Matthew Bower

Abbreviations

AD   Autosomal dominant
AR   Autosomal recessive
NGS   Next-generation sequencing
WES   Whole exome sequencing
WGS   Whole genome sequencing

Key Points
- While hereditary neuromuscular conditions most often follow distinct patterns of inheritance, clinicians should be aware of important exceptions to these patterns.
- There are many distinct ways in which DNA can be altered resulting in neuromuscular disease. Genetic testing technologies may have important limitations in detecting some specific types of alterations.
- Variant interpretation is a complex and evolving process. Clinicians should be aware that the classification of some specific variants is subject to change as we learn more about genetic variation both in health and disease.

Introduction

Recent advances in molecular techniques have led to the development of a vast array of molecular diagnostic tools for neuromuscular clinicians. While these new testing methods offer the promise of precision patient-centered management, the results often introduce additional uncertainties. In many cases, genetic test results may fail to identify a causative mutation in a patient with a clearly inherited

M. Bower, MS (✉)
University of Minnesota Health, Department of Genetic Counseling, Minneapolis, MN, USA
e-mail: MBOWER1@fairview.org

© Springer International Publishing AG, part of Springer Nature 2018   191
D. Walk (ed.), *Clinical Handbook of Neuromuscular Medicine*,
https://doi.org/10.1007/978-3-319-67116-1_10

condition, or testing may identify genetic variants of uncertain clinical significance. In order for the neuromuscular clinician to navigate the complexities and uncertainties of genetic testing, it is critical to have a basic understanding of human genetics and the benefits and limitations of available tests. This chapter provides a high-level overview of human genetics and genetic testing as it applies to the person with neuromuscular disease.

Clinical Utility of Genetic Testing

Before embarking on a genetic "diagnostic odyssey," it is important for the clinician and the patient to carefully consider the utility and limitations of genetic testing. Academic curiosity on the part of the clinician alone is not a sufficient rationale to order *clinical* genetic testing—testing which may incur a large financial bill for the patient and may not provide the patient with desired information. Clinicians should engage patients in a thoughtful discussion of the potential utility of genetic testing for diagnosis, prognosis, management, and family planning. Examples of the utility of genetic testing for all four include the following:

- *Diagnosis*: Establishing a precise diagnosis, particularly for patients with rare neuromuscular disease, traditionally involved a lengthy, costly, and invasive diagnostic odyssey. In some circumstances, gene testing may provide a specific diagnosis without the need for muscle biopsy, EMG, or other diagnostic procedures.
- *Prognosis*: Genetic testing may, in some cases, provide valuable prognostic information to patients and families. A salient example is a newborn infant with significant hypotonia. Molecular testing may help to clarify whether a neuromuscular condition is expected to follow a degenerative or static course. This in turn provides families with critical information needed to make decisions such as whether to continue or withdraw ventilator support.
- *Medical management*: Molecular diagnosis may facilitate optimal medical management for a given patient. In the case of limb-girdle muscular dystrophies, genetic testing can more precisely identify patients in need of additional cardiac screening [1]. In other cases, establishing a genetic diagnosis may preclude therapeutic trials of immunosuppression when both genetic and inflammatory etiologies are on the differential diagnosis list. Perhaps the most dramatic example is SMA, in which molecular diagnosis identifies patients who will benefit from gene therapy.
- *Family planning*: Genetic testing may provide important information for family planning. An individual with an autosomal recessive condition may rest assured that the risk of recurrence in his/her children is small, while a patient with an autosomal dominant disorder must consider a disease risk, depending upon penetrance, of up to 50% to each offspring. A precise genetic diagnosis facilitates the communication of risk to other family members and, more importantly, allows them to pursue options such as carrier testing, predictive testing, prenatal testing, and preimplantation genetic diagnosis. Such options are typically only available to a family if a precise genetic diagnosis has been established.

Genetic testing raises complex questions that are best addressed by a certified genetic counselor when one is available. Genetic testing requires informed consent and a clear explanation of its purpose and pitfalls. An excellent review of ethical considerations in genetic testing in neuromuscular disease is referenced here and highly recommended [2].

Genetics and Inheritance

The human genome is encoded by 3 billion bases of DNA spread across 23 pairs of chromosomes. The first 22 pairs of chromosomes are present in two copies in both males and females and are called "autosomes." The 23rd pair of chromosomes, the sex chromosomes, consists of the larger X chromosome and the much smaller Y chromosome. Females have two copies of the X chromosome, while males have a single copy each of the X and Y chromosomes. This difference in sex chromosomes is important for understanding X-linked inheritance, discussed below. In addition to the DNA contained in the 23 pairs of chromosomes, there is also mitochondrial DNA in every cell. Mitochondria, which are present in multiple copies in every cell, harbor their own independently inherited genomes.

Most clinical genetic testing focuses on the small proportion of DNA (approximately 2%) that encodes proteins. This small portion of coding DNA, collectively referred to as the *exome*, is believed to encode 20,000–25,000 genes, the majority of which have not yet been implicated in human disease. The exact function of the remaining noncoding DNA, which constitutes about 98% of the human genome, is largely unknown. For many years, this noncoding DNA was referred to as "junk" DNA, which most likely reflected a lack of understanding of its role. Recent systematic efforts have now assigned specific biochemical functions to more than 80% of this noncoding DNA [3]. These functions include, but are not limited to, expression of small RNA molecules, gene regulation through transcription factor binding, and mediation of chromatin structure through epigenetic modification, such as DNA methylation or histone acetylation. The principal structures of genetic material are illustrated in Fig. 10.1.

In 2003, the first draft of the human genome reference sequence was published. Since that time, the reference sequence has been updated multiple times. Most humans differ from the established reference sequence at millions of different positions, with most of this variation considered normal or benign. Variations from the reference sequence that cause disease are typically referred to as *mutations* or *pathogenic variants*. These mutations may be passed through families in one of several well-characterized patterns of inheritance: autosomal dominant, autosomal recessive, X-linked, or mitochondrial. Key features of these patterns are listed in Table 10.1 and Fig. 10.2. It is important to recognize that these features may not be universally present in every patient or family. In some cases, these features may not be present due to small family size or the patient's specific social situation (e.g., undisclosed adoption). Some important biological exceptions to the standard inheritance patterns, such as reduced penetrance and de novo mutations, are discussed in detail below.

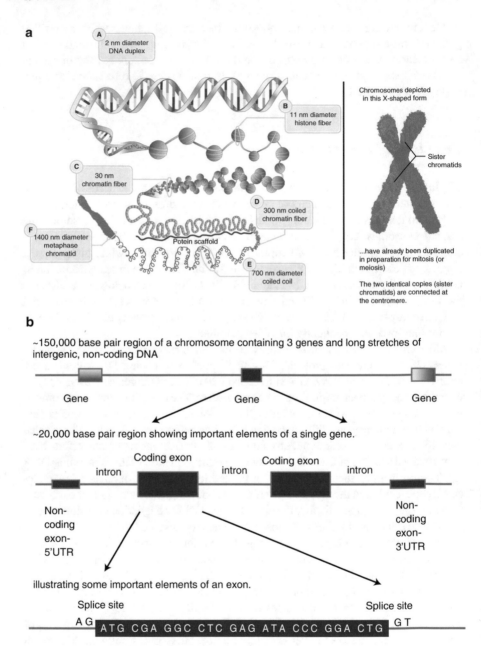

Fig. 10.1 (a) Overview of the structure of chromosomes and DNA. (b) Schematic drawing of the components of a gene

Table 10.1 Common patterns of inheritance

Inheritance pattern	Defining features	Examples
Autosomal dominant	Single mutation sufficient to cause disease Male-to-male transmission (not always present in every family) Presence of disease in multiple generations (unless mutation is de novo) Males and females similarly affected Risk to offspring of an affected individual is 50%	C9orf72-ALS Myotonic dystrophy FSHD CMT1A
Autosomal recessive	Two mutations (one on each allele) necessary to cause disease Affected individuals usually confined to a single sibship in a family Disease typically not present in multiple generations Risk to offspring of an affected individual is typically small	SMA
X-linked	Absence of male-to-male transmission Females typically unaffected carriers or more mildly affected than males Risk to offspring depends upon gender of offspring	Duchenne/Becker muscular dystrophy
Mitochondrial disease due to mutation in mt genome	Risk to offspring is dependent upon gender of affected parent Affected females pass mutation to all children Affected males do not transmit mutation to children Clinical phenotype highly variable and dependent upon percentage of mitochondria affected and tissue distribution of affected mitochondria	MELAS MERRF
Mitochondrial disease due to nuclear DNA mutation	Clinical findings and/or muscle biopsy findings suggestive of mitochondrial disease Family history fits one of the above patterns (e.g., male-to-male transmission suggesting dominant inheritance)	Mitochondrial DNA depletion syndrome due to POLG mutation

Inheritance Patterns

Autosomal disorders are caused by mutations in genes located on chromosomes 1–22 and are thus present in two copies in both males and females. Autosomal conditions typically affect both males and females equally. *Autosomal dominant* inheritance occurs when a single mutation is sufficient to cause the clinical phenotype. In such families, the disease is often, but not always, present in multiple generations. *Autosomal recessive* disorders, by contrast, require a mutation on both copies of the gene (one inherited from each parent). In such families, the disease is typically confined to a single sibship.

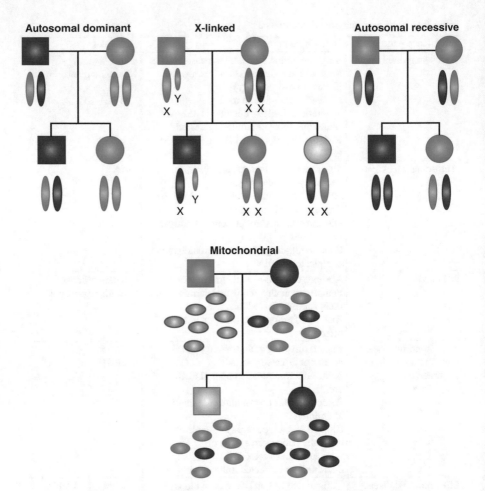

Fig. 10.2 Features of common inheritance patterns. Affected individuals are colored red, while clinically unaffected individuals are colored blue. Chromosomes containing a mutated gene are illustrated as red ovals below the individuals in the pedigree, while chromosomes containing a normal gene are illustrated as blue ovals. The autosomal dominant pedigree illustrates a male-to-male vertical transmission of the phenotype, which confirms autosomal dominant inheritance. The X-linked pedigree illustrates a female carrier of a mutation. Her offspring include an affected male, an unaffected noncarrier female, and a female carrier who may manifest a very mild clinical phenotype (light red) depending upon X-inactivation pattern. The autosomal recessive pedigree illustrates two unaffected carrier parents who have a single affected male child and an unaffected female carrier child. The mitochondrial pedigree illustrates a mother who carries a mitochondrial DNA mutation in a proportion of her mitochondria. She passes both normal and mutant mitochondrial DNA to all of her offspring. The proportion of mutant mitochondria, and resulting clinical phenotype, may vary significantly among her offspring

X-linked disorders are caused by mutations on the X chromosome. X-linked conditions preferentially affect males as they have only a single copy of the X chromosome. *Because males do not pass their X chromosome to their sons, the presence of "male-to-male" disease transmission in a family history excludes X-linked inheritance.* In some cases X-linked disorders may be developmentally lethal in males, in which case only affected females may be observed in the family. X-linked conditions may be classified as *X-linked recessive* when heterozygous females do not typically manifest clinical findings (e.g., DMD) or as *X-linked dominant* if heterozygous females typically manifest the disease in spite of the presence of a normal allele on the other X chromosome (e.g., Rett syndrome).

In rare cases, females who carry an X-linked mutation may manifest some or all of the features of an X-linked recessive disorder due to a phenomenon known as *skewed X inactivation.* Females typically silence or inactivate either the paternal or maternal X chromosome in each cell. This silencing is usually random and results in a mix of cells using either the maternal or paternal X chromosome. In some cases, this inactivation may be nonrandom or "skewed." If a disproportionate number of cells maintain an X chromosome with a detrimental mutation as active, a female may manifest some or all of the features of an X-linked disease.

*Mitochondrial diseases***:** Mitochondria are unique organelles in that they possess their own genome, which is inherited independently from the much larger nuclear genome. Each cell typically has thousands of mitochondria, each of which has its own mitochondrial genome and each of which may harbor its own DNA variants. The fact that each cell, and by extension each tissue, has a mixed population of mitochondria is referred to as *heteroplasmy.* Mutations in mitochondrial DNA may be present at a very low level across many different tissues. In other cases, mutant mitochondrial DNA may be present at a very high proportion in some tissues (e.g., muscle) while being nearly undetectable in other tissues (e.g., leukocytes). This varying distribution of mitochondrial DNA mutation burden explains in some part the wide clinical spectrum of mitochondrial disease and also the difficulty of identifying a pathogenic mutation in some cases.

Mitochondrial DNA is inherited in a unique pattern, termed *maternal inheritance.* While mitochondria are present in both the sperm and egg cells at conception, only maternal mitochondria (from the egg cell) persist through early development, while the paternal mitochondrial contribution (from the sperm cell) is lost. The precise mechanism by which the paternal mitochondrial contribution is lost has not been fully elucidated, and some rare exceptions of paternal mitochondrial inheritance have been reported [4]. As with all other cells, the egg cell contains a heterogeneous mitochondrial population. Thus, females with mitochondrial disease typically transmit a variable proportion of mutant mitochondria to each offspring. The precise burden of mutant mitochondrial DNA, to some extent, may predict the severity of disease in each offspring.

While the mitochondrial genome contains many of the genes necessary for mitochondrial function, a much larger proportion of mitochondrial genes are actually encoded in the nuclear genome. Thus, many mitochondrial diseases (those due to mutations in nuclear-encoded genes) actually follow the aforementioned nuclear patterns of inheritance (autosomal dominant, recessive, or X-linked).

Exceptions to the Mendelian Inheritance Patterns

When evaluating family history, neuromuscular clinicians should be aware of some exceptions to the aforementioned patterns of inheritance.

Anticipation is a phenomenon in which the age of onset becomes progressively earlier in each successive generation (Fig. 10.3). Anticipation occurs in a subset of trinucleotide repeat diseases and is related to the instability of the repeat sequence and growth in the size of the repeat between generations. The most notable example of anticipation for neuromuscular clinicians is myotonic dystrophy type 1. The presence of anticipation may complicate diagnosis in a proband as symptoms may not be present or formally diagnosed in other family members. Gender bias for these types of expansions is often noted, but these biases are not absolute. As an example, significant expansion of the CTG repeat associated with myotonic dystrophy type 1 most often occurs with maternal transmission [5] but may also occur with paternal transmission [6].

De novo mutations are mutations that occur at or near the time of conception and are thus not apparent in either biologic parent. In point of fact, the exact timing of the de novo mutation is almost never determined, which may have important implications for diagnostic testing in the proband and/or reproductive counseling of parents.

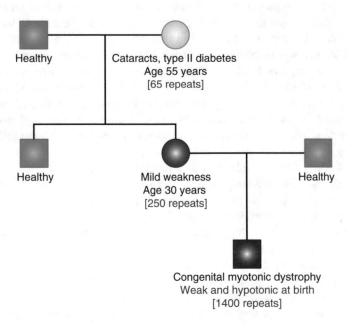

Fig. 10.3 The phenomenon of anticipation in a family with myotonic dystrophy type 1. CTG repeat numbers for each individual are given in brackets []. The family first came to attention with the birth of a child with the congenital form of myotonic dystrophy [1400 repeats]. Subsequent clinical evaluation of the mother revealed findings consistent with adult-onset myotonic dystrophy and a CTG repeat number of 250. The maternal grandmother had subtle findings that may not have been recognized as myotonic dystrophy and had only 65 CTG repeats

De novo mutations may arise in the germ cells of the transmitting parent. In this case, one would expect the mutation to be present in all tissues in the affected child, but they may not be detectable in blood samples in the parent. This may have important reproductive implications if a substantial proportion of parental germ cells harbor the mutation. One important situation that illustrates this is the case of the mother of an apparently sporadic (no prior family history) case of Duchenne muscular dystrophy. Even if the mother tests negative for the mutation in her blood, there is still a significant risk for having another affected child [7].

Mosaicism refers to situations where a de novo mutation arises post-zygotically in the developing embryo/fetus (Fig. 10.4). In this case, the mutation may not be present or detectable in all tissues. Mosaicism may be confined to a specific tissue type (e.g., muscle) while absent from other tissue types (e.g., leukocytes). In this situation, a pathogenic mutation could be missed unless the affected tissue is analyzed. In other situations, mutations may be present across multiple tissue types but at a level that is low enough to escape detection by traditional DNA testing techniques.

Reduced penetrance (Fig. 10.5) refers to situations where some mutation carriers do not manifest clinical findings during a normal life span. For some disorders penetrance is almost 100% (e.g., males with pathogenic dystrophin mutations), whereas for other disorders (e.g., facioscapulohumeral muscular dystrophy), a significant percentage of mutation carriers do not manifest clinical findings [8]. It is important to emphasize in such cases that while the clinical disease may not be present in all generations, the mutation itself does not "skip generations."

Precise estimates of disease penetrance are often difficult to derive as they may depend on several factors. For some disorders, age-specific disease penetrance is available. For example, approximately 50% of individuals with a pathogenic C9orf72 expansion would be expected to manifest ALS or FTD by age 50 [9], while penetrance is nearly complete by age 80 [10]. For other conditions, such as myotonic dystrophy, patients with very mild mutations may manifest only limited findings (e.g., cataracts) that may not be immediately apparent when reviewing the family history. For X-linked conditions such as Duchenne muscular dystrophy, the definition of penetrance in female carrier may vary depending upon whether one is referring to rare cases of fully manifesting females or more broadly speaking of females with subtle findings (e.g., mild muscle weakness or myalgias) [8].

Nonpaternity or undisclosed adoption: Patients report the family history as they believe it to be, which may or may not reflect true biological relationships in a family. Clinicians should be aware that misunderstood relationships could mask the presence of a dominant or X-linked disease in a family. Beyond the traditional issues of nonpaternity or undisclosed adoption, one must also consider the increasing frequency of in vitro pregnancies achieved with donor sperm or donor eggs—information which may or may not have been specifically disclosed to the child conceived with these methods.

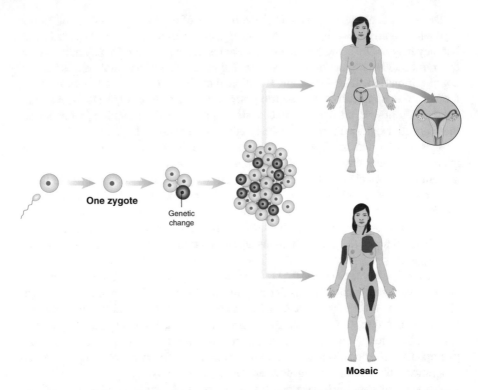

Fig. 10.4 Mosaicism. Following fertilization, a single-cell zygote rapidly grows through cell division. While each daughter cell typically contains the same DNA, mutations can arise in a single cell (pink cell). The descendants of this mutated cell can be distributed in a number of ways through the body. The top portion of the figure illustrates a situation where cells harboring the mutation are confined to the ovary (gonadal mosaicism). In this situation, the individual may not manifest clinical findings of the disease but can transmit the mutation to multiple offspring. The bottom portion of the figure illustrates a situation where the mutation is distributed throughout muscle tissue but is absent from the blood. In this latter scenario, a patient may be clinically affected with a neuromuscular disease, but the mutation may not be identifiable when analyzing the blood

Types of Mutations

Most DNA diagnostic testing focuses on the detection of small-scale changes in the genetic code, such as substitutions involving a single base pair or small deletions or insertions involving a handful of bases. Such changes are generally detected through methods that can be broadly categorized as "sequencing." DNA sequencing methods determine the base pair composition in the patient's DNA and then compare the patient's DNA sequence to an established reference sequence.

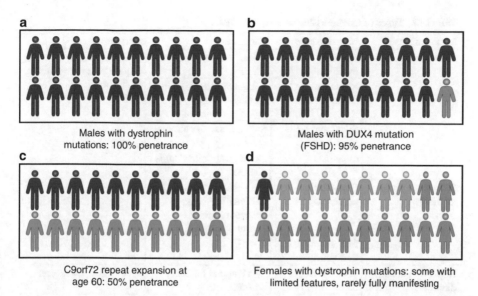

Fig. 10.5 Reduced penetrance in hereditary neuromuscular disease. Affected individuals are colored red and unaffected individuals are colored gray. (**a**) Males with a pathogenic dystrophin mutation demonstrate 100% penetrance of the disease phenotype. (**b**) Approximately 5% of males with a pathogenic D4Z4 contraction affecting DUX4 will not manifest a clinical phenotype of FSHD (95% penetrance). (**c**) Age-related penetrance in carriers of C9orf72 mutations. By age 60, only 50% of mutation carriers will manifest clinical disease. The penetrance increases with age and is nearly 100% by age 80 (not illustrated here). (**d**) Penetrance of neuromuscular phenotypes in female carriers of dystrophin mutations. A small number of females carrier may manifest frank neuromuscular disease. A larger percentage (light-red shading) will manifest mild phenotypes that may include muscle cramps and myalgias. The majority of female carriers are clinically silent

Variations from the reference are then interpreted. These methods will be discussed in more detail in the next section (Table 10.2).

Small changes in DNA sequence may exert their effect through a number of different mechanisms (Fig. 10.6):

Single-Base Substitutions

Single-base substitutions in coding DNA have one of three possible effects (Fig. 10.6a). First, a DNA substitution may alter the codon in which it occurs, leading to a change in the encoded amino acid. This type of substitution is termed a *missense* variant. Further evaluation is required in order to determine whether a given missense substitution is pathogenic or benign (discussed below). Second, DNA substitutions may change a codon to a stop codon, which is termed a *nonsense* mutation. With a small number of exceptions, nonsense mutations are predicted to result in a loss of protein function and would be considered pathogenic for diseases in which

Table 10.2 Types of mutations and detection methods

Mutation class	Mutation type	Example	Detection method
DNA substitution	Missense mutations	p.Leu276Ile (L276I) in *FKRP*	DNA sequencing of coding sequence and intron/exon boundaries
	Nonsense mutations	p.Arg894* (R894X) in *CLCN1*-related myotonia congenita	
	Silent mutations	Spinal muscular atrophy	
	Splice site mutations	GAA c.-32-13 T > G mutation in mild Pompe disease	
Small insertions/ deletions	Frameshift mutations	Frameshift mutations in *SLC5A7* in distal hereditary motor neuronopathy VII A	
	In-frame deletion or duplication	OPMD	
Repeat expansion disorders	Trinucleotide repeat expansion	DM1, spinal bulbar muscular atrophy	Fragment size analysis
	Other repeat expansions	DM2, C9orf72	Combination of methods including southern blot and/or PCR-based methods
Gross deletions/ duplications	Whole gene deletion or duplication	PMP22 deletions or duplications	Quantitative methods including MLPA, array CGH, qPCR, or NGS-based CNV detection
	Partial gene deletion or duplications	Partial DMD deletions or duplications in Duchenne muscular dystrophy	
Complex genomic rearrangements		FSHD	Specialized test methods including southern blot

loss of function is an established mechanism of disease. Finally, a DNA substitution may have no predicted effect on the encoded amino acid, a *silent* variant. While the majority of silent substitutions are expected to be benign, there are some very important exceptions—notably the silent substitution in exon 7 of SMN1 that can cause spinal muscular atrophy [11].

Single-base substitutions may also occur outside of the coding DNA and exert their effects through other mechanisms such as disruption of splicing. The most frequently identified noncoding substitutions involve the intronic DNA sequence immediately adjacent to the exon/intron boundary. This DNA sequence is highly conserved, and disruption of the sequence can either abolish or significantly disrupt normal splicing. Substitutions that alter splicing may also be identified in regions distant from the coding exons (deep intronic mutations). Deep intronic mutations may create new splice sites that significantly disrupt the normal protein structure. Deep intronic mutations are typically not evaluated by clinical tests as these types of variants are rare and difficult to functionally characterize.

Small Deletions or Insertions

Small deletions or insertions in the genetic code are often detected by the same methods that are used to identify the substitution mutations described above. There is no precise definition delineating "small" deletions/insertions from "large" deletions/insertions. Traditional sequencing methods can typically detect deletions or insertions smaller than 15–20 bp, although this threshold may vary significantly depending upon the specific laboratory protocols. Larger deletions that involve hundreds or thousands of bases of DNA typically require other methods for detection (see below).

Small insertions or deletions can be classified depending upon whether they involve a number of nucleotides that are a multiple of 3. If the insertion or deletion is a multiple of 3, then the consequence is the insertion or removal of amino acids in the protein (*in-frame mutation*). In some cases, these insertions or deletions may be well tolerated, while in other cases, they may result in significant clinical disease. Oculopharyngeal muscular dystrophy is an example of a relatively modest in-frame insertion causing a well-characterized neuromuscular disease [12].

Small insertions or deletions that are not a multiple of 3 nucleotides typically result in a *frameshift mutation* (Fig. 10.6b). Frameshift mutations disrupt all of the codons that occur downstream and typically result in either a complete loss of gene function or a grossly abnormal protein. The exact consequence of a frameshift mutation may depend on several factors including whether it occurs early or late in the gene, whether it introduces an early stop codon or extends the reading frame beyond the normal stop codon, and whether the resulting gene transcript is degraded or translated into an abnormal protein. In most cases, frameshift mutations result in a loss of function, but important examples of frameshifts resulting in gain of function have been reported [13].

Repeat Expansion Disorders

The importance of repeat expansion disorders was first appreciated in the early 1990s with the discovery of the genetic basis of fragile X syndrome, myotonic dystrophy type 1, and SBMA. These disorders involve repetitive stretches of DNA that vary in size in the normal population but can cause disease when they reach a critical size threshold (Fig. 10.6c). While these disorders share a common genetic mechanism (expansion of a repetitive DNA sequence), each disease has specific pathogenic repeat size. Broadly speaking, each of these diseases has a normal repeat range that is observed in the healthy population and does not cause disease or confer a significant risk of disease for subsequent generations. Each disease also has a pathogenic threshold beyond which point most or all individuals would be expected to manifest disease during a normal life span. In between these two ranges, there are often intermediate repeat numbers that may be of reproductive significance only, or of *possible* clinical significance. For many repeat expansion disorders, the size of

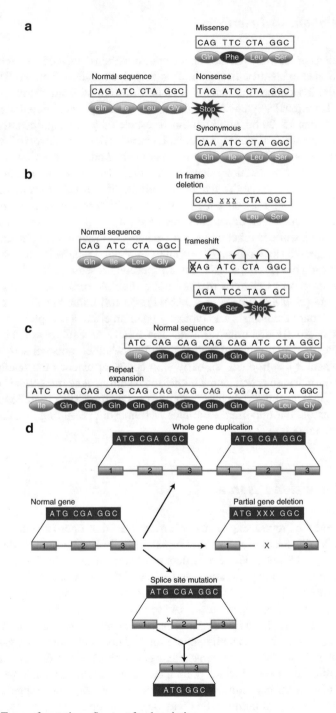

Fig. 10.6 Types of mutations. See text for description

the repeat expansion correlates with age of onset or clinical severity. Finally, as described above, some repeat expansion disorders may demonstrate anticipation in which the repeat size expands when transmitted, resulting in progressively younger age of onset with each new generation in a family.

Structural Variation

Structural variation refers to large-scale deletions, duplications, or rearrangements of the genetic code (Fig. 10.6d). For the sake of this review, such changes are defined as involving at least one entire coding exon of a gene, which is usually several hundred base pairs in length. *Structural variations are typically not evaluated by traditional DNA sequencing techniques and require specific quantitative methods for detection.* Structural variations may involve portions of a gene, an entire gene, or multiple contiguous genes. In some cases, it is sufficient to establish the presence of a genomic deletion or duplication for diagnosis. In other cases, additional structural information may be required. For example, in FSHD, it is sometimes necessary to demonstrate both the deletion of repeated D4Z4 sequences AND to establish that the shortened sequence resides on a permissive haplotype on chromosome 4 [14].

Genetic Testing Methods

A comprehensive discussion of molecular genetic testing methods is beyond the scope of this brief chapter. For many neuromuscular diseases (e.g., FSHD or SMA), specialized disease-specific methods have been developed. For more information about these methods as they relate to specific diseases, the reader is referred to www.genereviews.org.

For many other neuromuscular diseases, molecular diagnosis is accomplished through sequencing. *Sequencing* refers to methods that determine the base sequence of a patient's DNA, compare the resulting sequences to the reference, and identify differences (variants) in the patient's DNA that are pathogenic. Traditionally, DNA sequencing was accomplished by a method called *Sanger sequencing.* While Sanger sequencing provides highly reliable data, it cannot be scaled up in a cost-effective manner to analyze large numbers of genes. In 2010, massively parallel or *next-generation sequencing* was integrated into the testing menus of many clinical laboratories. Next-generation sequencing is a process in which a patient's DNA is fragmented, the resulting fragments are attached to a physical surface and sequenced, and the resulting sequence fragments are reassembled using complex computer algorithms. Next-generation sequencing technology provides the same type of sequence information as traditional Sanger sequencing but can be economically scaled for analysis of large numbers of genes.

Table 10.3 Rationale for targeted gene testing in selected neuromuscular diseases

Disease	Targeted test prior to broad-based testing	Proportion of mutations	Rationale
Charcot-Marie-tooth, demyelinating type	PMP22 duplication	43–63% of CMT patients who receive a molecular diagnosis	Large genomic rearrangements may not be routinely analyzed by NGS
Spinal muscular atrophy	Homozygous SMN1 deletion	95%	NGS methods may not accurately distinguish between highly homologous genes (SMN1 vs. SMN2)
Amyotrophic lateral sclerosis (ALS), familial	C9orf72 hexanucleotide expansion (CCCCGG)	20–30% of autosomal dominant ALS	Current NGS technologies cannot accurately assess large repetitive noncoding GC-rich sequences
Myotonic dystrophy, types 1 and 2	Trinucleotide expansion of DMPK (type 1) versus tetranucleotide expansion of ZNF9 (type 2)	100% of DM1 and DM2	Current NGS technologies cannot accurately assess large repetitive noncoding GC-rich sequences
Muscular dystrophy, childhood onset	Dystrophin (incidence of Duchenne MD, 1 in 3500 male births)	50–75% of pathogenic mutations are large deletions or duplications	Large genomic rearrangements may not be routinely analyzed by NGS
Facioscapulohumeral muscular dystrophy (FSHD), type 1	Genomic rearrangements involving D4Z4 repeat in 4q35	95%	Current NGS technologies cannot accurately assess large repetitive noncoding GC-rich sequences

One can think about methods in terms of a spectrum with targeted methods at one end (e.g., testing for the CTG repeat associated with myotonic dystrophy type 1) and broad-based methods at the other end (e.g., whole exome sequencing). Intermediate options (such as phenotype-specific multigene sequencing panels) often are available as a compromise between these two extremes. Each approach has benefits and limitations, and, in practice, a combination of approaches may be employed depending upon the specific clinical situation.

Targeted methods typically query a single locus or a limited number of loci in the genome (Table 10.3). From a practical standpoint, the benefits of choosing such an approach include minimizing cost, turnaround time, and incidental findings. Such methods are typically analyzing a limited number of loci where there is high-quality evidence correlating mutations with the clinical phenotype. The drawback of this approach is that if the common mutation(s) is absent, the testing does not provide information beyond the queried loci. These methods also may not be suited to situations where many genes cause the same or overlapping phenotypes, limb-girdle muscular dystrophy being a salient example.

In contrast, broad-based methods may query many genes simultaneously, some of which may have very limited evidence to support a correlation with clinical disease. Broad-based genetic testing, such as whole exome sequencing, has been employed as a "second step" once high-likelihood diagnoses have been excluded by targeted testing. The rationale for this is threefold. First, targeted testing often represents the quickest and most cost-effective way to establish a precise diagnosis. This remains true for many conditions, such as myotonic dystrophy. Second, employing targeted tests as frontline tests reduces the likelihood of generating information that is uncertain or not desired by patients. Finally, in spite of the "comprehensive" promise of whole exome sequencing, this technology has several important technical limitations. For example, whole exome sequences cannot evaluate repeat sequence length (e.g., myotonic dystrophy and C9orf72-related ALS), may not identify large-scale genomic changes (e.g., FSHD), and may not correctly analyze genes with highly similar copies in the genome (e.g., SMN1 and SMN2 in spinal muscular atrophy).

In between these two extremes are phenotype-driven multigene panels. These panels often represent a diagnostic compromise between the two extreme approaches and may be the first-line approach in cases where mutations in one of several genes may cause clinically overlapping phenotypes.

Recently, broad-based methods have gained traction as the primary diagnostic test in certain clinical situations, particularly in cases where a patient's clinical presentation does not fit with a well-described clinical phenotype [15]. In such cases, a patient may represent a very atypical presentation of an established clinical disease. In other cases, it is now well known that many patients with "atypical presentations" may have more than one Mendelian diagnosis [16]. In such cases, a patient may benefit from the unbiased approach of broad-based testing. In other situations, such as when patient's insurance may only cover a single round of genetic testing, it may be in the patient's financial interest to pursue the most comprehensive test available as the first-line test.

Variant Interpretation

The ease with which large amounts of DNA can be queried has created a new problem in genomics—how to interpret the increasing number of rare and novel variants identified in patients. Until recently, this interpretation process was not standardized, and the same DNA variant in the same patient might receive discordant interpretations depending upon which laboratory was performing the testing.

The American College of Medical Genetics and Genomics and the Association for Molecular Pathology issued a joint guidance in 2015 in an attempt to standardize the process for variant interpretation [16]. In addition to providing a vocabulary for describing the clinical significance of DNA variants (benign, likely benign, uncertain significance, likely pathogenic, or pathogenic), these guidelines established and weighted the types of evidence to be used in variant interpretation. While this has standardized the variant interpretation process across laboratories, discordant variant interpretations remain a significant problem [17].

Population data are among the first-line tools used by laboratories to determine whether or not a variant should be interpreted as pathogenic or benign. Some laboratories with expertise in testing specific genes may have accumulated variant data from large numbers of patients tested for those genes. These databases may be proprietary or may be publically available. These databases may provide the frequency of rare alleles in patients with the disease in question.

Other databases are intended to represent the genetic diversity in the general population. The largest of such databases that are publically available is the Genome Aggregation Database (gnomAD) from the Broad Institute, with exome data from over 125,000 individuals and whole genome data from an additional 15,000 individuals at the time of this writing. While the curators of gnomAD have attempted to remove individuals with severe pediatric diseases, one must exercise caution in assuming that all of the individuals in such a large database are "healthy controls."

When querying such databases, clinicians are typically posing the question: *Is the variant sufficiently rare to cause the disease in question?* A variant that is present in 1:1000 individuals is too common to be the cause of a rare fully penetrant autosomal dominant disease that affects 1:100,000 individuals. One must be careful in drawing conclusions in cases where a disease is not fully penetrant, where the age of onset is late enough that a clinical phenotype may not have been apparent at the time the database was assembled or the clinical phenotype is sufficiently mild that an individual would not have been excluded from a control database. In addition, population databases cannot claim to represent all human genetic diversity, and caution is urged in using these databases to interpret variants found in patients whose ethnic background may not be well represented in current databases. Links to relevant population databases are provided in the appendix.

Locus or disease-specific databases are catalogs of variation in specific disease-causing genes. These include large public databases, such as ClinVar and the Leiden Open Variation Database, and commercial databases available to subscribing customers such as the Human Gene Mutation Database (HGMD). Other locus-specific databases may be individually maintained by specific scientists, clinicians, or institutions. A catalog of other locus-specific databases is available through the Human Genome Variation Society. Users should be aware that these databases may contain both benign and pathogenic variants. Ideally these databases include both a clinical assertion for a variant (e.g., pathogenic or benign) AND the data used to support this conclusion. It is incumbent upon the neuromuscular clinician to critically review the supporting evidence to determine whether it supports the clinical assertion for the variant. Links to relevant locus-specific databases are provided in the Appendix.

Peer-reviewed publications are an important source of information for variant interpretation. Publications should be read with a skeptical eye, and the actual evidence provided in the publication should be subjected to critical review. Older publications may have determined that a particular variant was pathogenic because it was "absent from controls," in which case it is important to establish how many controls were evaluated. It was not uncommon for a "control data set" in the pre-genomics era to only include 50–200 individuals. Additional evidence included in publications may include whether the variant segregated with the phenotype in the family, whether the variant arose "de novo" in the affected individual, and whether a functional consequence of the variant was verified using an in vitro method or animal model. Ideally, the neuromuscular clinician should extract this evidence and determine whether or not it is sufficient to conclude that the variant is pathogenic.

In silico models are computational tools used to predict the consequences of mutations. Each tool makes a prediction based upon specific factors such as conservation across species or biochemical properties of the involved amino acids. Other in silico models provide predictions of how a particular variant may impact splicing. *These models are considered the weakest evidence in variant interpretation* [16]. While these models may provide supportive evidence, conclusions about pathogenicity should not be based primarily upon these models.

Epigenetics

Epigenetics refers to heritable traits that result from factors other than changes to the DNA sequence. These types of changes include methylation of specific bases or chemical modifications of the DNA-binding proteins (histones) resulting in changes in gene expression (Fig. 10.7). Epigenetic modification of DNA may arise due to inherited changes in DNA sequence, may be influenced by environmental exposures, or may be reset or altered depending upon the gender of the transmitting parent. There are some discrete examples of inherited epigenetic changes causing disease such as Prader-Willi syndrome and Angelman syndrome. The region of chromosome 15 associated with these syndromes undergoes differential methylation depending upon whether the chromosome is inherited from the mother or the father. Biparental inheritance of this region is required for normal development. Molecular testing for Prader-Willi syndrome and Angelman syndrome evaluates for the presence of both maternal and paternal epigenetic markers in this region. While epigenetic changes likely play an important role in other neuromuscular diseases, as of this writing, there are few situations in which testing for epigenetic status serves as a primary diagnostic tool.

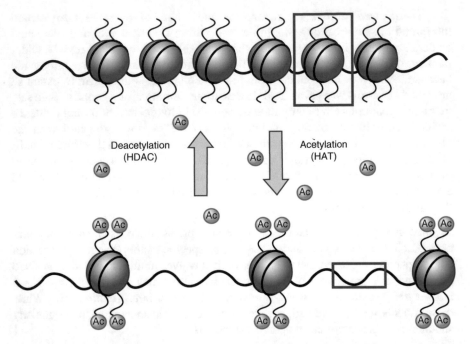

Fig. 10.7 Epigenetic modifications. (**a**) The top strand of DNA illustrates DNA in an inactive conformation. The DNA is tightly wrapped around histones (purple circles), and genes are unavailable to the transcription machinery. (**b**) Epigenetic modifications, such as acetylation of histones, relax the DNA into an open conformation. This allows genes (red box) to be expressed

Conclusion

Molecular genetic testing is a powerful diagnostic tool for the neuromuscular clinician. The benefits of this testing are best realized in the context of a thoughtfully obtained clinical and family history and thorough clinical examination. While the costs and technical barriers continue to fall, interpretive challenges will remain for many years to come. As new evidence emerges, variants previously categorized as having uncertain clinical significance may be recognized as pathogenic. Alternatively, variants previously suspected of causing disease are often recategorized as benign based upon information from larger and more comprehensive population databases. Therefore, it is incumbent upon the neuromuscular clinician to keep up-to-date on developments in this field and critically evaluate and periodically re-evaluate results of all genetic testing.

Additional Resources

Gene reviews is a collection of expert-authored and peer-reviewed clinical synopses of inherited conditions. At present, there are 679 "chapters" each focused on a specific genetic disease or phenotype.

- https://www.ncbi.nlm.nih.gov/books/NBK1116/

Human Genome Variation Society nomenclature guidelines: This website has published standard mutation nomenclature guidelines used to accurately describe DNA, RNA, and protein variants in databases, clinical reports, and publications. In addition, this website has links to locus-specific databases that are maintained independently of ClinVar and LOVD.

- www.hgvs.org
- http://varnomen.hgvs.org/

Genome Aggregation Database (gnomAD): Allele frequencies in control database comprised of >140,000 individuals. This is the largest publically available database of its type. At the time of this publication, this resource was still under development.

- http://gnomad.broadinstitute.org/

Exome Aggregation Consortium (ExAC): This is the predecessor to gnomAD, with exome data from >60,000 individuals. Much of the data are being rolled into the larger gnomAD database, but ExAC currently has some data not yet available in gnomAD such as exon-level copy number variation data.

- http://exac.broadinstitute.org/

ClinVar: This is a public database of variants and clinical assertions (pathogenic vs. benign). Submissions may be accompanied by varying types and amounts of evidence supporting the clinical assertion.

- https://www.ncbi.nlm.nih.gov/clinvar/

Leiden Open Variation Database is similar to ClinVar but based in Leiden University in the Netherlands. Data are organized by specific genes. The Leiden database has a long history of cataloging normal and pathogenic variation in neuromuscular disease genes.

- www.lovd.nl

References

1. Narayanaswami P, Weiss M, Selcen D, David W, Raynor E, Carter G, et al. Evidence-based guideline summary: diagnosis and treatment of limb-girdle and distal dystrophies. Neurology. 2014;83:1453–63.
2. Su X, Kang PB, Russell JA, Simmons Z. Ethical issues in the evaluation of adults with suspected genetic neuromuscular disorders. Muscle Nerve. 2016;

3. ENCODE Project Consortium. An integrated encyclopedia of DNA elements in the human genome. Nature. 2012;489(7414):57–74. https://doi.org/10.1038/nature11247.
4. Schwartz M, Vissing J. Paternal Inheritance of Mitochondrial DNA. N Engl J Med [Internet]. 2002;347(8):576–80. Available from: http://www.nejm.org/doi/abs/10.1056/NEJMoa020350
5. Rakocevic-Stojanovic V, Savić D, Pavlović S, Lavrnić D, Stević Z, Basta I, et al. Intergenerational changes of CTG repeat depending on the sex of the transmitting parent in myotonic dystrophy type 1 [2]. Eur J Neurol. 2005;12(3):236–7.
6. Bergoffen J, Kant J, Sladky J, Mcdonald-mcginn D, Zackai EH, Fischbeck KH. Paternal transmission of congenital myotonic dystrophy. J Med Genet. 1994;31:518–20. Original articles
7. Vanessen AJ, Busch HFM, Temeerman GJ, Tenkate LP. Birth and population prevalence of Duchenne muscular-dystrophy in the Netherlands. Hum Genet. 1992;88(3):258–66.
8. Zatz M, Marie SK, Cerqueira A, Vainzof M, Pavanello RCM, Passos-Bueno MR. The facioscapulohumeral muscular dystrophy (FSHD1) gene affects males more severely and more frequently than females. Am J Med Genet. 1998;77(2):155–61.
9. Majounie E, Renton AE, Mok K, Dopper EGP, Waite A, Rollinson S, et al. Frequency of the C9orf72 hexanucleotide repeat expansion in patients with amyotrophic lateral sclerosis and frontotemporal dementia: a cross-sectional study. Lancet Neurol [Internet]. 2012;11(4):323–30. Available from: https://doi.org/10.1016/S1474-4422(12)70043-1
10. Benussi L, Rossi G, Glionna M, Tonoli E, Piccoli E, Fostinelli S, et al. C9ORF72 hexanucleotide repeat number in frontotemporal lobar degeneration: a genotype-phenotype correlation study. J Alzheimer's Dis [Internet]. 8(4):799–808. Available from: http://content.iospress.com/articles/journal-of-alzheimers-disease/jad131028. 2014 Jan 1 [cited 2017 Jun 27].
11. Monani UR, Lorson CL, Parsons DW, Prior TW, Androphy EJ, Burghes AH, et al. A single nucleotide difference that alters splicing patterns distinguishes the SMA gene SMN1 from the copy gene SMN2. Hum Mol Genet [Internet]. 8(7):1177–83. Available from: http://www.ncbi.nlm.nih.gov/pubmed/10369862. 1999 Jul [cited 2017 Jun 26].
12. Brais B, Bouchard JP, Xie YG, Rochefort DL, Chrétien N, Tomé FM, et al. Short GCG expansions in the PABP2 gene cause oculopharyngeal muscular dystrophy. Nat Genet [Internet]. 18(2):164–7. Available from: http://www.nature.com/doifinder/10.1038/ng0298-164. 1998 Feb [cited 2017 Jun 26].
13. Barwick KES, Wright J, Al-Turki S, McEntagart MM, Nair A, Chioza B, et al. Defective presynaptic choline transport underlies hereditary motor neuropathy. Am J Hum Genet [Internet]. 91(6):1103–7. Available from: http://linkinghub.elsevier.com/retrieve/pii/S0002929712005290. 2012 Dec 7 [cited 2017 Jun 26].
14. Lemmers RJLF, O'Shea S, Padberg GW, Lunt PW, van der Maarel SM. Best practice guidelines on genetic diagnostics of Facioscapulohumeral muscular dystrophy: workshop 9th June 2010, LUMC, Leiden, The Netherlands. Neuromuscul Disord [Internet]. 22(5):463–70. Available from: http://linkinghub.elsevier.com/retrieve/pii/S0960896611013423. 2012 May [cited 2017 Jun 26].
15. Fogel BL, Satya-Murti S, Cohen BH. Clinical exome sequencing in neurologic disease. Neurol Clin Pract [Internet]. 6(2):164–76. Available from: http://cp.neurology.org/lookup/doi/10.1212/CPJ.0000000000000239. 2016 Apr [cited 2017 Jun 26].
16. Richards S, Aziz N, Bale S, Bick D, Das S, Gastier-Foster J, et al. Standards and guidelines for the interpretation of sequence variants: a joint consensus recommendation of the American College of Medical Genetics and Genomics and the Association for Molecular Pathology. Genet Med [Internet]. 17(5):405–24. Available from: http://www.nature.com/doifinder/10.1038/gim.2015.30. 2015 May 5 [cited 2017 Jun 26].
17. Amendola LM, Jarvik GP, Leo MC, McLaughlin HM, Akkari Y, Amaral MD, et al. Performance of ACMG-AMP variant-interpretation guidelines among nine laboratories in the Clinical Sequencing Exploratory Research consortium. Am J Hum Genet [Internet]. 98(6):1067–76. Available from: http://linkinghub.elsevier.com/retrieve/pii/S0002929716300593. 2016 Jun 2 [cited 2017 Jun 26].

Index

© Springer International Publishing AG, part of Springer Nature 2018
D. Walk (ed.), *Clinical Handbook of Neuromuscular Medicine*,
https://doi.org/10.1007/978-3-319-67116-1

Printed in the United States
By Bookmasters